HEALING
SMOOTHIES

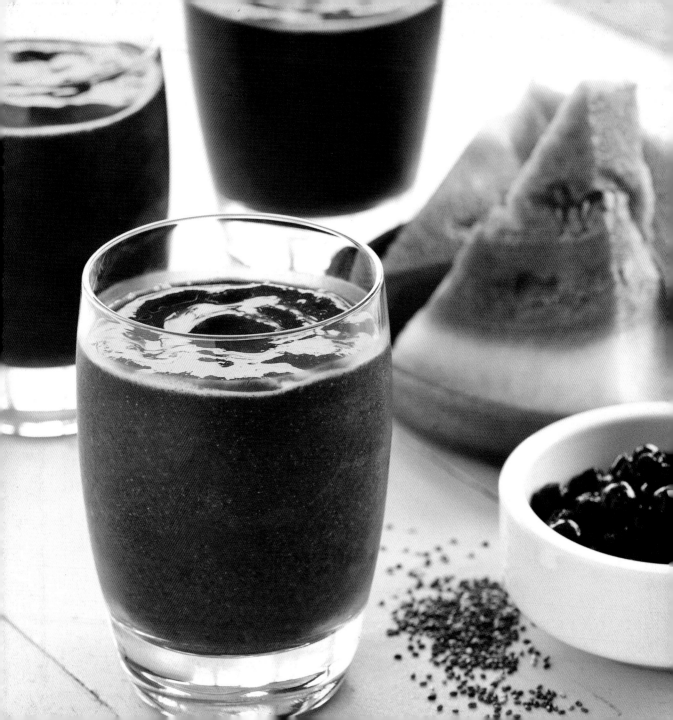

HEALING
SMOOTHIES

100 Research-Based, Delicious Recipes That
Provide Nutrition Support for Cancer Prevention and Recovery

Daniella Chace, MSc, CN

From the author of the bestselling *More Smoothies for Life* and
What to Eat if You Have Cancer

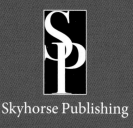

Skyhorse Publishing

Skyhorse Publishing books may be purchased in bulk at special discounts for sales promotion, corporate gifts, fund-raising, or educational purposes. Special editions can also be created to specifications. For details, contact the Special Sales Department, Skyhorse Publishing, 307 West 36th Street, 11th Floor, New York, NY 10018 or info@skyhorsepublishing.com.

Skyhorse® and Skyhorse Publishing® are registered trademarks of Skyhorse Publishing, Inc.®, a Delaware corporation.

Visit our website at www.skyhorsepublishing.com.

10 9 8 7 6 5 4 3 2

Library of Congress Cataloging-in-Publication Data is available on file.

Cover design by Erin Seaward-Hiatt
Cover photos by Olivia Brent

Print ISBN: 978-1-63220-447-9
Ebook ISBN: 978-1-63220-759-3

Printed in China

This book is dedicated to my assistant Helen Gray, who is one of my oldest friends. Her dedication to the details around the editing, product research, and photography allowed me to focus on the clinical and culinary development of this book.

Contents

Introduction

As a clinical nutritionist specializing in the burgeoning field of oncology nutrition in the late '90s, I was in charge of developing the nutrition protocols for an integrative cancer clinic in Seattle. This was a challenging assignment as cancer creates specific nutritional needs. My patients were exhausted and overwhelmed by food planning, shopping, and preparation. There were other considerations as well, such as the side effects of treatment that affect appetite. For example, the nausea caused by chemotherapy can be triggered by the smell of cooked foods.

Early in my career as a nutritionist I co-authored *Smoothies for Life*, which is a functional recipe book with smoothies that provide health benefits such as sleep improvement, energy enhancement, and weight loss. I began to apply my experience in creating medicinal smoothies to resolve some of the dietary issues of my patients, including alleviating chemo-induced nausea and inflammation.

Then I set to work researching each of the specific nutrients my patients needed such as carotenoids, probiotics, fiber, essential fatty acids, and protein, and finding the highest quality foods that provide these nutrients. This involved considering the importance of organic, whole foods while avoiding Genetically Modified Organisms (GMOs), allergens, processed foods, and toxins. I created smoothies for patients, often designing them to meet individual needs, which meant addressing dietary restrictions, cost, and availability.

Making fresh smoothies daily can become an enjoyable practice. This simple routine can be adhered to for years and, in turn, the medicinally active nutrients provide protection and healing benefits that increase over time.

I have learned from years of observation that daily smoothies can dramatically improve energy during treatment and the outcome of treatment. Smoothies can provide proper nutrition throughout treatment, reduce the length of time that treatment is needed, and when the daily smoothie routine is maintained after treatment, reduce the chance of recurrence in the future.

Misinformation on the Internet
Much of what we see online and via website bloggers is inaccurate and misleading. I'm disheartened when I read popular websites with outdated and blatant misinformation about oncology nutrition. Even some of the trusted websites linked to television programs aren't thoughtful or informed in their discussions and recommendations about food and cancer. The guidance in this book comes from decades of working with cancer patients and thousands of evidence-based studies.

Effective Therapy
Smoothies are easy to whip together, and also provide powerful nutrient therapy. There is a tremendous amount of nutrition and toxicology research to consider when developing food recommendations for medical conditions. I first must calculate the daily dose of the nutrients in the studies to apply to smoothies. Then I spend weeks in the kitchen developing recipes that contain these specific nutrients at concentrated enough levels to provide benefits. The finished product is a collection of medicinally active, nutrient-rich smoothies made from fresh whole foods.

Bioactive Anticancer Nutrients
The ingredients in these recipes provide powerful nutrients to support healing and remission. I chose each of these food nutrients for their direct action against cancer such as improving signaling pathways, reducing angiogenesis (reducing blood flow to cancer cells), increasing energy, reversing cachexia (muscle loss), inhibiting the inflammation that can lead to cancer, and triggering apoptosis, which is the programmed destruction of cancer cells.

Empirical Research

The information and recommendations provided here are all based on research conducted by reputable academic and clinical institutions. The studies used as the basis for these recommendations are available in the References section in the back of the book and at daniellachace.com.

Medical Nutrition Therapy

The following have been developed to provide a high concentration of healing nutrients while also accommodating most dietary restrictions. The recipes are vegan, gluten-free, high in protein, and devoid of common allergenic foods including dairy, soy, corn, and wheat.

Synergistic Ingredients

Many of the ingredients have been chosen for the synergistic effects of their nutrients, for example, black pepper's ability to increase the effectiveness of curcumin.

Metabolically Active Nutrients

The nutrients in these smoothies must also be highly absorbable so that they can be absorbed by the intestines, received in the bloodstream, and delivered to the cancerous cells. Consider, for example, how anthocyanins have the ability to reduce the inflammation that drives cancer but only when first metabolized by gut flora. To incorporate these elements into a smoothie, we not only need anthocyanin-rich foods such as berries, but we also need probiotics such as those found in cultured coconut milk.

Laboratory Studies

Translating medical research into dietary recommendations is difficult because many studies are done in a laboratory setting, with mice, or using extracts rather than whole foods. The link between specific food nutrients and how they change the development of cancer is clear. However, how much we need to ingest and how often is not as clear. We do know that eating foods with specific nutrients consistently and frequently will benefit us over time. When possible, I have used the dietary percentage information directly from the corresponding research in order to calculate the dosage (amount of that food) needed to provide the benefits found in the study.

Oncology Nutrition Research

Over the last few years there has been a tremendous surge in research identifying the specific nutrients that have the ability to change the course of cancer.

There is more oncology research being done around the world than ever before. With a clearer understanding of the role that food nutrients, toxins, and microflora play in disease prevention and development we have reached some long-sought answers to our questions about what triggers, promotes, heals, and prevents cancer. There is direct evidence showing us the toxins and nutritional deficiencies that create the environment for cancer cell development.

This research provided the basis for the following recipes. These nourishing infusions support those in treatment and those who aim to nourish their bodies to prevent the development or recurrence of cancer.

Epigenetics

There have been great advances in the field of epigenetics, which is the study of the nutrients and toxins that can influence gene expression. There was a long-held belief that genes had a permanent plan for our biology. We now know that even if we have a genetic marker for cancer it will not necessary be "expressed" and that we can, via epigenetics, effect whether that gene will direct our cells to develop cancer.

Specific nutrients and toxins can turn cancer cells off and on. For example, piperine, a nutrient compound found in black pepper, has an epigenetic effect. This means that it can reduce the expression of specific cancer genes, even ones that are programmed for cancer. Researchers have found that piperine may be a potential agent for the prevention and treatment of human breast cancer as it reduces HER2 overexpression.

Even though this is a new science, the research so far strongly indicates that individuals can benefit from applying what we know to date about nutrients and toxins in epigenetic therapy.

The Microbiome
We also have the exploding field of human microbe research, which has shown us that our bodies are living laboratories of health-supporting bacteria. These organisms play a key role in nutrient metabolism and immune regulation. For years we were confounded by conflicting results from nutrient studies. We now understand that the unknown variable was microbes. When we have a healthy level of these symbiotic gut flora, we can absorb cancer-healing nutrients such as anthocyanins, but without them many nutrients are useless to us.

From Research to Dietary Recommendations
Cancer incidence is increasing. With so much at risk, it is critical that we translate this new research into useful dietary recommendations as it is made available. Yet, much of the research published in medical journals has not made its way into the mainstream as daily recommendations, as part of oncology protocols, and as a primary support to cancer patients.

Smoothies provide an easy and direct way to start incorporating these cancer-fighting nutrients into our recovery plans immediately.

Who Should Use This Book

Daily smoothies promote recovery for those who are in treatment as well as providing protection from recurrence for those in remission.

Those with either a known family history of cancer, or genetic tests indicating a propensity for it, can benefit from these smoothies that contain nutrients that affect genetic expression. Learn more about epigenetics and cancer at daniellachace.com.

Those in remission can also benefit as many of the nutrients in these smoothies have been found to reduce the risk for cancer recurrence.

Individual Response to Food Nutrients
Keep in mind that we each respond differently to various foods, nutrients, treatments, etc. Cancer develops when we have a combination of imbalances that allow abnormal cells to run amok. While one person may have a reduction in cancer cells from ingesting food nutrients, another person's cancer may respond more directly to the removal of toxins, such as BPA, for example.

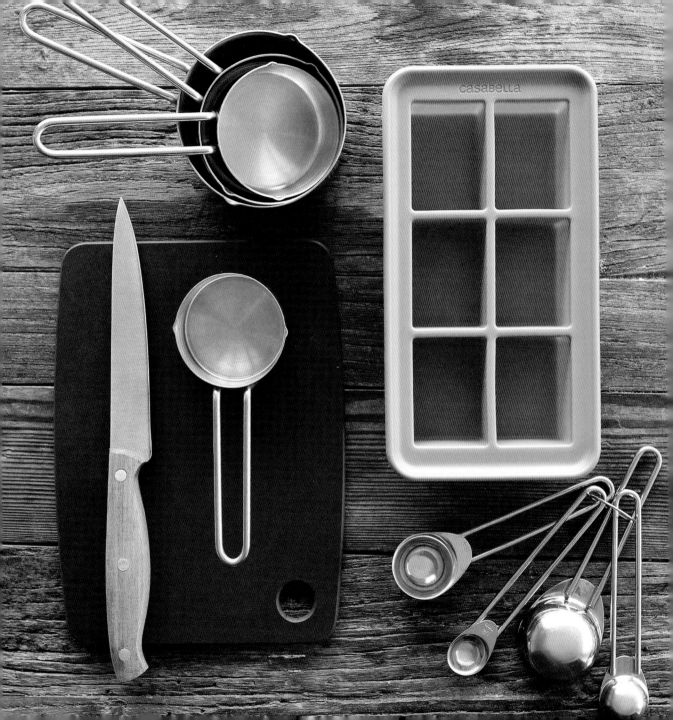

How to Use This Book

These smoothie recipes are designed to provide nourishing support for patients throughout both the healing process and remission. The recipes contain nutrients proven to support the healing process including protein, vitamins, minerals, antioxidants, and essential fatty acids. Food nutrients have many effects that can prevent and inhibit the process of cancer; they can increase our white blood cells' ability to react to cancer cells, reduce blood flow to cancer tissues, turn off genetic signaling pathways, and cause apoptosis, which is literally the destruction of existing cancer cells.

In general, a cancer-recovery diet is one that is low in sugar and contains no synthetic compounds such as chemical sweeteners, colorings, preservatives, or plastic residue from packaging. A cancer-recovery diet is also one that is anti-inflammatory and contains minimal phytoestrogens (plant estrogens), which could potentially stimulate hormone sensitive cancers.

Most of the ingredients are widely available at grocery stores, but a few of the ingredients may not be available in your local market. For those ingredients, a visit to a natural foods store or a quick search online should turn up the items you're seeking.

At the end of each recipe I've included a reference to the most relevant study supporting the use of a particular nutrient in the recipe. The References section in the back of the book provides a list of the current cancer research on each food nutrient I've recommended.

The How to Make a Smoothie section outlines the basic steps to making successful smoothies. The Kitchen Tools section covers the essential equipment needed for smoothie-making and how to choose non-toxic tools.

Non-Toxic Ingredients

Many of the so-called healthy drinks at the store and in restaurants actually promote cancer cell growth. For example, many are high in sugar, which suppresses the immune system and feeds cancer cells. These drinks often contain phthalates from the plastic containers used to ship their ingredients, which can stimulate the growth of hormone-sensitive cancers.

Making smoothies at home allows you to use the highest quality ingredients with minimal chemical exposure.

Metabolically Available Nutrients

Probiotics support nutrient metabolism, so adding ingredients like cultured coconut milk or probiotic supplements to smoothies is recommended in order to increase the bioavailability of the food nutrients you're consuming.

The Smoothie Ingredients section (page 26) is a more involved list that provides information about how to prep each ingredient—for example, removing the rind from melons and removing the pits from stone fruit and cherries.

Medicinally Potent Ingredients

I want to emphasize that the research, upon which my recommendations are based, strongly indicates that these nutrients, when ingested daily, can fuel the body's defense against cancer in specific and powerful ways, such as reducing the risk of development, inhibiting the growth, reducing metastasis, causing apoptosis, and reducing existing cancerous tumors.

Daily Smoothie Infusions

Making smoothies part of your daily routine is one of the easiest ways to practice good nutrition and actively support the healing process each day.

These nutrient-dense drinks can be added to your current diet. For example, you may want to drink one first thing in the morning, have another smoothie for a snack during the day, and a third as a dessert in the evening.

Drink between one and four of these smoothies daily to continually infuse your body with their benefits. Cells divide constantly and can divide in either a healthy or unhealthy way. The nutrients found in these smoothie recipes will promote healthy cell development most effectively when they are taken consistently.

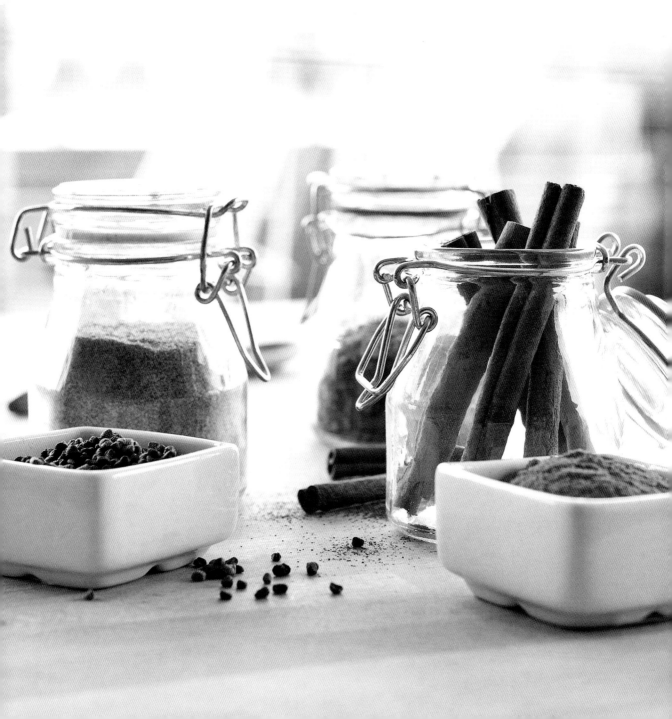

Nutrition Guidelines for Cancer Healing Smoothies

Create Customized Smoothies

Once you've tested some of the various combinations, you might find that there are certain flavors that you like best. Using your personal taste preferences, you can begin to customize your own recipes.

For example, I use a lot of frozen fruit because I love the texture of frosty drinks. However, if your blender struggles to macerate frozen foods, or if you just prefer fresh or thawed produce, there is no need to add frozen items to your smoothies.

Use these recipes as a guide to the many foods that promote healing from cancer. I've included a variety of foods and arranged them in the amounts and combinations that I find most appealing. However, it is not necessary to replicate a smoothie exactly as it is in the book. Feel free to use your favorite juice, fruit, and protein. For example, if you don't want to buy vanilla beans, leave them out or use vanilla extract.

The following list provides the basic nutritional guidelines for creating your own healing smoothies at home.

Increased Protein Needs

Dietary protein is needed for immune function, wound-healing, and fighting fatigue. Many of us don't get enough protein on a daily basis and cancer increases our need for protein by up to 25 percent. By adding a concentrated source of protein to each smoothie you will be able to easily meet your daily requirement.

When we are at our healthiest, we need between 50 and 100 grams per day depending on our life stage and activity level. When we have cancer, we need approximately 65 to 125 grams of protein per day.

Besides protein powder supplements, there are several high-protein ingredients that work well in smoothies—for example, chia seed and hulled hemp seed blend well. They are also rich in omega-3 fatty acids that help reduce inflammation.

Reducing inflammation is important as evidence suggests that inflammation may cause a majority of the fatigue felt during and after treatment. Hulled hemp seed and chia seed are not only rich in omega oils but they are also whole-food, vegan, and often organic.

Low Sugar
Keep the sugar content of your smoothies as low as possible. Sugar feeds cancer cells, suppresses the immune system, and increases inflammation, bacteria, and fungus. Avoid sweeteners such as table sugar and fructose. Even natural sweeteners such as maple syrup, agave, and honey should be avoided.

And keep in mind that synthetic sweeteners such as aspartame and Splenda should be avoided even though they don't have carbohydrates (sugar). Many of these synthetic sweeteners cause a host of problems including joint pain and headaches.

Nutrient-Rich Ingredients
Plant foods contain nutrients such as antioxidants that play a key role in healing cancer. By incorporating foods rich in these nutrients into your daily smoothies, you are ensuring that they are available as needed for your body's healing processes.

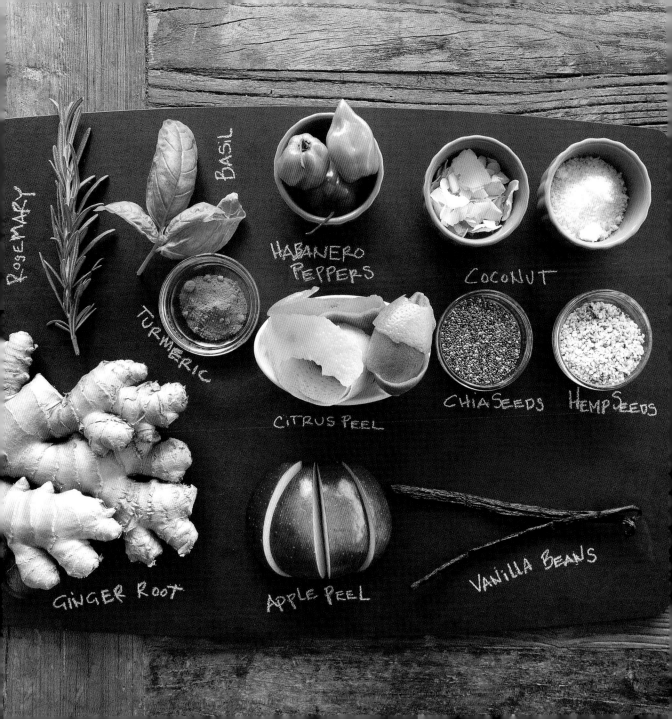

ROSEMARY

BASIL

HABANERO PEPPERS

COCONUT

TURMERIC

CITRUS PEEL

CHIA SEEDS

HEMP SEEDS

GINGER ROOT

APPLE PEEL

VANILLA BEANS

Hormone Safe EFAs

Healthy, non-toxic, vegan sources of essential fatty acids that are free of phytoestrogens, which pose a risk for certain types of breast cancer, are primrose oil, borage oil, hemp seed, and chia seed.

Avoid Plastic

Avoid plastic food containers when possible as most contain phthalates including bisphenol A (BPA), diethyl phthalate (DEP), and dibutyl phthalate (DBA), which have been implicated in scientific studies as causative factors in the development and growth of certain types of cancer.

We don't know the effects of the newer "BPA-free" plastic containers until they can be studied further, so it is safer to use stainless steel or glass food and water containers until we know more.

Organic is Non-Toxic

Many pesticides and herbicides are carcinogenic. Buy organic when possible and keep a list of the produce that is most heavily sprayed so you will be able to choose organic when it matters most. For example, strawberries are heavily sprayed, which means it's important to buy organic strawberries. For a list of produce that is the least sprayed, see EWG.org.

Minimize Soy

Soy foods contain phytoestrogens, which have been suspected of stimulating hormone-sensitive cancer growth. Study results have been inconsistent, which may be due to the natural, person-to-person variance of both gut flora and nutrient absorption. Microbes in the intestine break down and release plant estrogens from certain foods such as soy, flaxseeds, and yams. Until we know more about estrogenic foods, it is best to avoid them.

Avoid Dairy

Dairy foods have been found to increase insulin-growth factor (IGF-1) levels, which have been linked to an increase in the growth of certain types of cancer.

Also milk and other dairy products have varying levels of certain hormones that have the potential to act as active hormones in our bodies.

The cancer risk from dairy may be caused by the genetically engineered bovine growth hormone, which is commonly injected into dairy cows to increase milk production. Preliminary studies show that organic dairy may be safe for breast cancer patients. However, until we have more evidence it is safest to avoid dairy altogether.

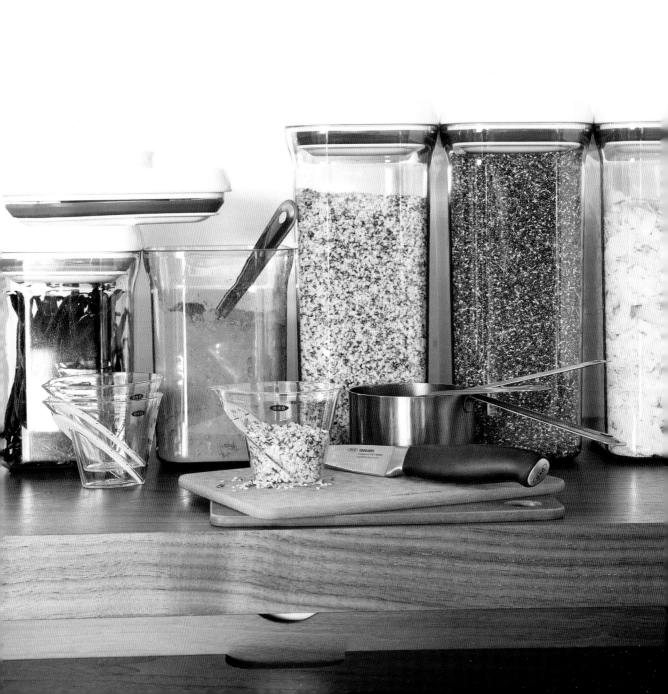

Kitchen Tools

Essential Kitchen Gear
The basic equipment needed for smoothies is a blender, a sharp knife, and a non-toxic cutting board. Besides those key tools, you may also want to have a spatula for scraping down the sides of the blender, a few silicone ice trays for making frozen tea cubes, waxed paper bags for storing fruits in the freezer, and a measuring cup and measuring spoons.

The Non-Toxic Kitchen
Buying non-toxic kitchen tools is important because heavy metals and plastics may cause cancer cells to grow and spread. Use glass, not plastic cups for serving your drinks. There are many well-designed, non-toxic kitchen tools these days making it easier than ever to set up a clean kitchen for smoothie making.

Blenders
The most important smoothie kitchen tool is, of course, the blender. High-power blenders are those that are over 700 watts.

Avoid plastics when possible by opting for a blender with a glass or stainless steel pitcher. If you have a blender with a plastic pitcher you can use it for cold drinks but avoid blending hot foods, which can leach plastic into the food. For example, avoid pouring hot tea directly into a plastic blender pitcher. Instead, brew the tea and let it cool. Then pour the cooled tea into the blender pitcher. Another option is to pour the tea into silicone ice cube trays to freeze for later use.

Even though some of these high-power plastic blenders have a heat function, I do not recommend using heat with plastic, especially prolonged heat.

The TriBest blender is a small, single-serve blender that fits well in tiny kitchens. It's tiny and powerful. It has a small base and uses glass mason jars as the pitcher. If the pitcher breaks, you can use any mason jar with their adapters as a replacement. Dual-use kitchen tools such as a mason jar blender pitcher also saves space in the cupboard.

If your current blender has a plastic pitcher, you may be able to replace it by using an adapter with a large mason jar as they fit most blender blade designs. Look online for demonstration videos to show you how this works.

Cutting Boards

Cutting boards are often made from toxic plastics. Over time the surface develops abrasions that release bits of plastic into the food. Instead of plastic or wooden boards, which harbor potentially dangerous bacteria, use pressed paper such as Epicurean brand cutting boards. They are non-toxic, last for years even with daily cleanings in the dishwasher, look great, and won't dull knives as fast as harder cutting board materials.

Knives

A high-quality knife is an important tool as it allows you to chop and prep produce quickly without a lot of mess or frustration. A quality knife is one that is made out of material that retains its edge without having to be sharpened weekly. Having at least one high-quality knife can reduce your time in the kitchen. Some prefer a small paring knife, but I use an eight-inch chef's knife for almost all of my chopping and slicing. Preparing produce is much easier with a sharp and sturdy knife.

Always hand-wash your knives; the dishwasher will dull them more quickly over time.

Measuring Tools

Glass or stainless steel measuring cups and spoons are non-toxic alternatives to the plastic varieties. Avoid other types of metal-coated tools as they often shed tiny bits of metallic material, contaminating food with toxic metals as they wear over time.

Spatulas
Choose high-heat resistant silicone spatulas such as Epicurean brand, which are non-toxic, resistant to heat as high as 500 °F / 260 °C, and dishwasher safe.

Food Storage Containers
Dry foods such as nuts and oatmeal can be stored in BPA-free plastic containers such as OXO Good Grip pop containers. Dry foods do not break down the plastic material, so there is little risk of food contamination from phthalates. I use them for my ground and shredded coconut, hulled hemp seed, chia seed, tea leaves, and nuts.

Save glass juice and jelly jars to reuse for storing liquids or buy glass containers with plastic lids (which don't touch the food) to store liquids.

Waxed paper bags or BPA-free bags can be used for freezer items rather than plastic food storage bags.

Water Filter
If possible, install a water filter (preferably a solid carbon or reverse osmosis filtration system) at your tap to remove chlorine, heavy metals, and other environmental contaminants from your drinking and ice cube water.

How to Make a Smoothie

There are just a few basic steps to making a successful smoothie.

1. Shop
Review the recipes you will be making for the week—check your refrigerator, freezer, and fruit bowl to see which ingredients you already have on hand. Then make a shopping list for those you will need to purchase at the store or online.

2. Prep
Prepare your produce by removing pits, washing, and chopping as necessary. Make frozen tea cubes or other items that need to be done ahead of time. The Ingredients section provides purchasing, preparation, and storage details for each ingredient.

3. Combine
When you're ready to make your smoothie, place your ingredients in the blender or food processor. First add liquids, then soft ingredients such as fruits and vegetables. Then add tougher and drier ingredients such as seeds, protein powder, and spices. Adding liquid first reduces pressure on low-power blender motors.

4. Blend
Blend the ingredients to your desired consistency. Frozen ingredients may bog down the blender motor. If this happens, add a little water and let the frozen ingredients thaw for a minute or two before blending.

5. Clean
Rinse the blender pitcher and put it away, or run it through the dishwasher to thoroughly clean the spaces around the blades and base.

Ingredients—Purchasing, Preparation, and Storage

Most produce requires little prep beyond a rinse before adding it to your smoothie. The General Preparation Tips below cover some of the most commonly asked questions.

The ingredient list can be used for a reference as it provides tips on how to identify, locate, purchase, prepare, and store each ingredient.

The ingredients on this list were chosen because they provide powerful and specific benefits for preventing and healing cancer. More detailed nutrient information is covered throughout the recipe section of this book and the research is provided in the references section.

General Tips

Organic Matters

Certain fruits and vegetables are heavily sprayed with herbicides and pesticides. Look for the USDA Organic label; foods carrying this label are not sprayed with these toxic chemicals. Also visit EWG.org for lists of the least and the most heavily sprayed produce.

Avoid Plastic

Look for juice sold in glass rather than plastic bottles. The acidity of the juice can break down the plastic interior of the bottle and leach toxic chemicals into the juice. Glass containers are non-toxic, and a safer option. Also look for juice labels that say 100% juice; this means the juice contains no added sugar or synthetic sweeteners. It is also possible to make your own juice at home with whole fruits and vegetables in a juicer.

Waxed paper bags or BPA-free food storage bags work well for storing frozen tea cubes and fruit in the freezer.

Juice, Tea, and Coconut Water Cubes

Coconut water, juices, and other liquids that will not be used within a few days of opening can be frozen for use in smoothies as ice cubes. Pour the liquid into stainless steel or silicone ice cube trays. Once the liquid is frozen, simply pop out the cubes into food storage bags where they will stay fresh in the freezer for months. This trick works equally well for brewed tea and fruit juices. I use frozen tea in many of my smoothies, so I measured the amount of liquid it takes to make ice cubes in my particular trays to get a better idea of how much frozen liquid I am adding with each ice cube. My ice cube trays make large ice cubes, and when I measured them I found that two cubes is equal to ¼ cup, so when I want ½ cup of green tea ice cubes, I know I can drop four cubes into my blender and there is no guesswork.

Smoothie Cubes

Leftover smoothies can also be frozen in ice cube trays. If you have leftover smoothies or just want to make them ahead of time, you can pour smoothies into ice cube trays, freeze them, then pop the cubes into freezer bags as described above and store them in the freezer.

The smoothie cubes can be dropped into a glass of water for a refreshing, nourishing and quick "smoothie fix" when you don't have time to blend a fresh drink. Smoothie cubes can also be blended with liquids such as chilled green tea, juice, or water.

You may want to prep this way for yourself when you have medical treatments planned or just busy days ahead. By doing a little prep work ahead of time you can stay on your smoothie program during days when you're tired or busy. Family and nurse providers will also find that this is the easiest way to keep up with the constant nourishment needs of those in their care.

Fresh Versus Frozen
There's nothing quite so wonderful as fresh fruit. However, many types of fruit remain at peak ripeness only a few days before they must be discarded. Therefore, frozen fruit is an easy alternative. Most fruit that we use in smoothies is available in the freezer section of the grocery store. Frozen fruit is prepped (for example, cherries are pre-pitted) and then frozen when it is in its prime. Store-bought frozen fruit is flash-frozen, which means the nutrient levels are comparable to those in fresh fruit. This modern freezing technique also prevents the fruit pieces from clumping together, making them easier to pour out of the bag.

Freezing Fresh Fruit at Home
If you have a surplus of fresh-picked or store-bought fresh produce that might not get eaten before it becomes overripe, you can freeze it. Prepare the fruit for freezing by removing the pit, seeds, or rind as described below for each item. When freezing berries, rinse them and let them dry well on a clean towel so they are dry when frozen, which keeps them from clumping.

Storing Leafy Greens
Fresh greens, such as kale and cilantro, have a short shelf life. But they can be kept fresh for several days. Rinse them; wrap them in a wet, clean towel; and store them in the refrigerator's crisper drawer.

Smoothie Ingredients

Apples
Fresh whole apples last for many weeks in a cool place such as the refrigerator or the garage. Prepare your apple by removing the core and stem. Apples that have been chopped can be stored in a covered glass container for up to a week in the refrigerator.

Applesauce works well in smoothies and is high in both fiber and many of the nutrients found in fresh, whole apples. However, because applesauce does not contain the skin of the apples, it is not as nutritious as unpeeled apple chunks. Nevertheless, it can be an apt addition to a smoothie as it contains quercetin, fiber, and antioxidants. Look for unsweetened applesauce in glass jars.

Organic, unfiltered apple juice in glass containers provides many cancer-fighting nutrients without the potential exposure to phthalates that are inherent in plastic bottles. Fresh apple juice can be made at home with a juicer, but this step is not necessary as most blenders and food processors make a quick slurry from whole apples.

Apricots
In the United States, fresh apricots are available in the produce department of most grocery stores during the summer months. The pit must be removed but the skin can be blended. Look for 100% apricot juice (also called apricot nectar) in glass bottles.

Bananas
Bananas are an ideal ingredient as they lend a creamy texture to the smoothie. When frozen, they give the smoothie a frosty, milkshake-like consistency. Bananas can be peeled and then frozen in food storage bags. Once frozen, bananas remain fresh for several weeks.

Banana peel has been found to contain anticancer compounds and it is edible when organic. Non-organic banana skins imported to the United States are toxic and should be avoided as they are saturated in pesticides.

Basil

Live sweet basil plants can be grown in a pot on the porch, in a sunny window indoors, or in outdoor gardens in warm climates. Fresh basil leaves are available in the produce department of most grocery stores and dried basil leaves are sold in bulk and in spice jars. Fresh and dried basil can be used in smoothies. Fresh is preferable as it has aromatic, healthful oils that provide more concentrated nutrients, flavor, and fragrance than dried basil leaves.

Beets

Beets are sweet, rich in carotenoids, widely available, and can be added raw to smoothies. Raw beets blend easily in high-power blenders and are preferable to canned beets as cans are often lined with toxic plastics. If you have cooked beets on hand they can also be used in smoothies but cooking isn't necessary if you're blending with a high-power blender.

Black Cherry Juice

Cherry juices and cherry concentrates are rich in nutrients and provide concentrated flavor in small quantities. Just ¼ cup of cherry juice provides sweet cherry flavor and fragrance to an entire smoothie. Buy organic cherry juices and concentrates when possible. Juices stay fresh for up to two weeks once opened and must be refrigerated.

Blackberries

Fresh or frozen blackberries can be added to smoothies for their flavor and nutrients. When picking fresh berries, be sure to rinse them well. Let them dry before freezing to avoid clumping and then store them in the freezer in food storage bags. Once frozen, they will keep for several months.

Black Pepper
Dried black peppercorns can be found in jars and in bulk in the spice section of the grocery store. Use a pepper mill to grind the peppercorns as needed. Grinding them will release their well-preserved, nutrient-rich oils.

Blueberries
Blueberries are such an ideal smoothie ingredient that they are sold in bags in the freezer section of most grocery stores specifically for smoothies. Fresh blueberries can also be used, or bought fresh and then frozen.

Wild blueberries are smaller, richer in flavor, and have a higher antioxidant content than common blueberries (see Wild Blueberries below).

Cantaloupe
Cantaloupe are a delicious addition to smoothies and can be added fresh or frozen. Just remove the rind and add the melon flesh, including the seeds. Fresh melon can be stored for months in an airtight container in the freezer. High-power blenders can easily blend frozen melon chunks, which give smoothies a frosty texture.

Cardamom
Cardamom pods and ground cardamom powder can be purchased from the bulk section of the grocery store. They give a heady aroma and flavor to smoothies and can be stored for up to a year in an airtight glass container.

Carrots
Whole fresh carrots can be blended in high-power blenders or fresh carrot juice can be added to smoothies. Carrot juice can be made at home with a juicer or purchased in the refrigerator section of the grocery store.

Chia Seed

Chia seed is rich in protein and essential fatty acids. These tiny seeds can be purchased at the grocery store or online. They blend well and act as an emulsifier. Chia seed can be added directly to smoothies or ground in a coffee grinder, which results in a powder that dissolves seamlessly when blended. Whole chia seeds and chia seed powder can be stored in an airtight container in the freezer for months.

Cherries

Pre-pitted, frozen cherries are ready to add to smoothies. Choose your favorite variety whether dark, sour, sweet, or tart as they all provide an array of immune-supporting nutrients. Buy organic when possible. If you're using fresh cherries, be sure to remove the pits. Once the pits have been removed, you can freeze them for future use. Cherry juice and cherry juice concentrate also contain most of the nutrients found in the whole fruit and a small amount adds intense cherry flavor to smoothies.

Tart cherries, tart cherry juice, and tart cherry juice concentrate contain bioactive compounds that have been found to trigger apoptosis in cancer cells when consumed frequently. Whole cherries must be pitted. Frozen cherries come pre-pitted and are generally frozen at the peak of ripeness so they're very sweet and easier to digest than unripe cherries.

Cilantro

Cilantro leaves have an intense flavor that most people either love or hate. I happen to love it. But these tiny, oil-rich leaves change the flavor of a smoothie quickly, so add just a tablespoon at a time and taste your blend before adding more so you can adjust the flavor to your palate.

Cinnamon

Ground cinnamon adds nutrients, a punch of flavor, and a little heat to smoothies. Buy it in glass spice jars or from the bulk department of the grocery store. Replace your cinnamon at least once a year as the oils oxidize when exposed to light and oxygen, causing it to lose both its health properties and flavor over time.

Citrus

Citrus fruits including oranges, grapefruit, tangerines, lemons, and limes contain powerful anticancer nutrients in their pulp, juice, and peel. They also add fresh fruit flavor and fragrance to smoothies.

Citrus peel has been found to contain concentrated amounts of anticancer compounds and is edible when organic. However, too much in a blender can bog down the blades and add an intense bitter flavor from the oils in the skin.

As a general rule, citrus fruits should be peeled before blending unless you use a high-power blender, in which case a small amount (about two tablespoons) of peel can be added.

High-power blenders can easily pulverize a few wedges of unpeeled or partially peeled citrus fruit. The white, pithy part of the peel is the part of the fruit that contains much of the bioflavonoids so leave as much of it on as possible.

Unpeeled fruit can be kept fresh in a cool dry place for up to a week. Peeled fruit can be stored in food storage bags in the refrigerator for about three days or in the freezer for months.

Citrus juice can be made at home or found pre-made in the grocery store. Citrus juice can be extracted from whole citrus fruit by cutting the fruit in half, poking the tines of a fork into the juicy part of the fruit, and twisting the fork to squeeze out the juice.

Pre-made, organic, 100% grapefruit, lemon, lime, orange, or tangerine juice is available in glass bottles in the grocery store. Santa Cruz and Lakewood are brands that sell organic citrus juice in glass. Fresh juice stays fresh in the refrigerator for weeks.

Cocoa

Unsweetened cocoa powder provides nutrients and rich chocolate flavor without sugar. Look for organic, unsweetened cocoa powders. I consider this a staple smoothie ingredient, especially if you're a chocolate fan. Unsweetened cocoa powder turns a smoothie into a chocolate treat that is rich in healing nutrients.

Coconut

Shredded unsweetened coconut is sold in the bulk department of many co-ops and grocery stores. It is naturally sweet. Sweetened coconut products should be avoided due to their sugar content. Coconut is available as a fine macaroon ground product that blends well in smoothies. Bob's Red Mill brand offers a range of coconut products, some finely ground and some coarsely shredded.

Coconut Milk

Coconut milk is a creamy, low sugar, gluten-free and vegan, dairy alternative. It's available in cartons that don't need refrigeration until opened, which makes them easier to store. You can buy a case and keep it in the pantry, which won't use up precious refrigerator space.

Coconut Water

Coconut water is the clear liquid from inside young coconuts and has a light coconut flavor. It is an ideal liquid base for smoothie making as it is low calorie, vegan, gluten-free, contains electrolyte minerals, and is especially rich in potassium.

Use coconut waters that are organic, to ensure the coconuts have not been sprayed with toxic chemicals.

Cranberries

Cranberry juice and cranberry juice concentrates add intense flavor and color to smoothies. Look for pure 100% cranberry juice with no added sweeteners in glass bottles.

Cultured Coconut Milk

Cultured coconut milk is actually much more like yogurt than milk and is vegan. It's sold in yogurt containers and is thicker than milk but not as thick as yogurt. I use So Delicious brand because it's unsweetened and organic. It is sold in tubs just like yogurt rather than milk cartons and found in the refrigerator section of the grocery store.

Cultured coconut milk contains probiotics, which provide the much needed microbes that help us metabolize our food. We need these organisms in our gut to help us absorb nutrients such as antioxidants.

Garlic

Garlic contains sulfide compounds that cause the breakdown and removal of cancer cells. Garlic has a strong flavor and scent, so start with one clove, blend, and taste. If you want more garlic flavor, add another clove and work your way up to your preferred level of heat and garlic bite. Peel garlic cloves before adding to a smoothie.

Fresh garlic is available year-round in the produce department of the grocery store. Dried garlic granules and dried garlic powder are also available in the spice and bulk sections of the grocery store. However, fresh is preferable because the oils in the cloves lose some of their medicinal properties when dried.

Ginger

Whole, fresh ginger root is found in the produce section of the grocery store. Ginger root juice, pickled slices, and ground ginger root powder can be used in smoothies. High-power blenders can pulverize the woody tuber and papery outer skin of fresh ginger root. However, if your blender has a hard time with tough fibers such as this, you can extract the juice by squeezing chopped fresh ginger root through a garlic press.

Grapes

Many of the nutrients in grapes are in the fruit's skin, so whole seedless grapes are ideal smoothie ingredients. Dark-colored grape juice, especially unfiltered, contains more of the nutrient-rich skin pulp. Buy organic when possible. Organic seedless grapes can be used fresh or stored in an airtight container in the freezer. Frozen grapes create a frosty and rich texture in smoothies.

Grapefruits

(See Citrus)

Green Tea

(See Tea)

Greens

Dark leafy greens including kale, baby spinach, cilantro, chard, and Italian parsley contain carotenoids such as lutein and zeaxanthin that provide protection against cancer cell development. Buy organic greens when possible as they contain higher levels of fat-soluble vitamins than non-organic greens.

Holy Basil

Tulsi, which is also known as holy basil, is a dietary herb used for its multiple beneficial pharmacologic properties including immune boosting and anticancer activity. Fresh holy basil leaves are available in the produce department of many specialty markets, farmer's markets, and ethnic markets. Live basil plants are often available at garden stores and can be grown in your own yard or in a pot on the porch.

Dried holy basil is available from the bulk spice section of many grocery stores. The dried leaves can be added directly to smoothies or, if your blender has a hard time breaking down dried herbs, they can be ground first in a coffee grinder. Holy basil powder can be stored in an airtight container in the freezer for months.

Hulled Hemp Seed
Hemp protein powder or hulled hemp seed products are vegan and rich in protein and omega fatty acids. They can be purchased in most stores and online. Bob's Red Mill line of products contains both, and they are always fresh and widely available. However, the powdered hemp products are often a little gritty and bitter. The whole hemp hearts, on the other hand, blend so well in smoothies that they create a cream-like texture. Overall, I find hulled hemp hearts to be fresher, nuttier, and more delicious than the powdered alternative.

Kale
Fresh kale leaves pair well with apples, lemons, and other citrus fruits. Buy organic kale when possible as organic greens contain higher levels of fat-soluble vitamins.

Lemons
(See Citrus)

Limes
(See Citrus)

Mandarin Oranges
(See Citrus)

Mangos
Mango flesh contains mangiferin, a bioactive xanthonoid that protects many types of cells from cancerous development. Remove the skin and pit before adding the sweet yellow flesh to your smoothie. Frozen mango, which has been peeled, pitted, chopped, and frozen, is available in the freezer section of the store. Since mangos may be genetically modified, it's important to buy organic.

Oats

Rolled oats provide cancer-preventing dietary lignans. Bob's Red Mill brand offers both organic and gluten-free rolled oats that can be purchased online and in most grocery stores.

Oranges

(See Citrus)

Papaya

It's possible to use the entire papaya in a smoothie. However, in my smoothies, I choose to cut away the skin and remove the seeds before using the flesh. Use fresh or freeze the chunks to give smoothies a rich, frosty texture. Lime pairs exceptionally well with this tropical fruit. Since papayas are often genetically modified, it's important to buy organic.

Peaches

Peaches are a stone fruit, so remove the pit before blending. The skin is edible. Once pitted, the fruit can be frozen to extend its shelf life. Stone fruits are heavily sprayed with agricultural chemicals. Buy peaches that are labeled "organic," which ensures that no chemical sprays have been used in the growing of the fruit.

Pineapple

Pineapple is sweet and has a tropical flavor. Fresh pineapple can be purchased in the produce department of most grocery stores. When shopping for a pineapple, smell the bottom of the fruit; a perfectly ripe pineapple will have a strong pineapple scent and its leaves should release easily when plucked. To prep fresh pineapple, use a knife to remove the skin, as well as about an inch off the top and the bottom, then slice the whole fruit. The fresh fruit can then be added to smoothies or frozen for future use. Canned pineapple is available but not recommended as the nutrient-dense core has been removed and the cans are lined with plastics that release phthalates into acidic foods such as pineapple.

Plums

Fresh plums are sweet and contain polyphenols that have the ability to trigger apoptosis in human cancer cells. Plums must have their pit removed before blending. The skin will blend easily and the pitted fruit can be frozen.

Pomegranates

Whole pomegranates are available seasonally in the produce section of the grocery store. The nutrients are contained in the pomegranate seeds, which are also known as arils. The whole fruit can be expensive and the seeds, which contain the juice, need to be removed from the fruit to be used in smoothies. Pre-frozen bags of pomegranate arils (a.k.a. seeds) are much easier to work with and are available in the freezer section of the grocery store. Organic 100% pomegranate juice and pomegranate juice concentrate are available in glass jars. The juice stays fresh for about a week once opened, but lasts much longer if frozen into cubes.

Probiotic Powders

Acidophilus and bifidophilus powders are sold in the bulk department of many co-ops and health food stores and multiple-organism probiotic capsules are available in most grocery stores.

Protein Powders

Organic and vegan protein powders are an excellent source of protein. They also help to thicken and emulsify smoothies. Look for pea or rice protein powders. Those with hormone-sensitive types of cancer may want to avoid soy and whey protein powders as they may contain plant and animal hormones, respectively.

Plain, unflavored protein powders are generally low in sugar. Read the label to make sure you aren't getting too much sugar when you opt for a flavored protein powder.

Prunes

Prunes are simply dried plums. The advantage of using dried plums rather than fresh is that they have a longer shelf life. They are pitted before they're dried so they're ready to add to smoothies, no preparation required. Prunes add sweetness, flavor, fiber, and active compounds that help reduce certain types of tumors.

Raspberries
Fresh raspberries need only be rinsed before adding to smoothies. Red raspberries are available in bags in the freezer section of the store.

Black raspberries can be picked fresh and can also be ordered online. Black raspberries are rich in polyphenolic anthocyanins, which have been shown to protect against the development of certain types of cancer by influencing the genes associated with inflammation.

Rosemary
Fresh, dried, and ground rosemary can all be used in smoothies. Fresh rosemary contains concentrated amounts of phenolic compounds that reduce inflammation and inhibit cancer cell growth.

Strawberries
Fresh and frozen strawberries provide sweet, fresh flavor and pink color to smoothies. Strawberries are a highly sprayed crop so it's essential to buy organic strawberries or grow your own. Fresh, organic strawberries should be rinsed and the green top can be removed and then added whole to smoothies.

Sunflower Seeds
Sunflower seeds provide protein, dietary lignans, and blend easily to create a rich texture and nutty flavor. Nuts and seeds can be stored in the refrigerator in an airtight container to reduce exposure to light and oxygen, which causes rancidity. They stay fresh for months when frozen.

Tangerines
(See Citrus)

Tart Cherries
(See Cherries)

Tea
Tea has a heady aroma and flavor. Brew loose leaf or bagged tea following the package instructions. Steep the tea for just under two minutes. By removing the leaves from the brewed tea at this point, you retain the maximum amount of protective catechins without extracting undesirable components like bitter tannins and excess caffeine. Let it cool before adding it to smoothies. Decaf tea can also be used as it provides all of the same nutrients as caffeinated tea but without the stimulating caffeine.

Brewed tea can be poured into ice trays to make frozen tea cubes. The cubes can be popped out of their trays, tossed into food storage bags, and placed in the freezer for quick use in smoothies. I prefer freezing tea because the cubes last indefinitely in the freezer and they add a frosty texture to smoothies.

Many teas including black, green, white, and spearmint have been found to reduce the risk for the development and recurrence of many types of cancer.

Green tea is tea made from the leaves of the tea plant, Camellia sinensis, that have not been oxidized by sun and light by the traditional process used to make black tea.

Green tea contains polyphenols such as epigallocatechin gallate (EGCG), which have anticancer activity. These nutrients provide protection from the development of cancer by reducing cell growth and genetic damage.

Herbal teas are those that are made from herbs and spices, and do not contain caffeine as do black, green, and white teas.

White tea comes from the buds and leaves of the Camellia sinensis plant, which contain concentrated amounts of the anticancer nutrient catechins and polyphenols.

Tomato
Fresh organic tomatoes of all varieties provide carotenoids that reduce oxidative stress. Organic tomatoes have a higher concentration of these nutrients than non-organic. Whole tomatoes can be added to smoothies. They pair well with citrus and greens.

Turmeric
Turmeric powder contains concentrated amounts of curcumin, which is effective in reducing inflammation and fatigue. Turmeric powder is made from the turmeric root. It is available in jars and in the bulk spice section of the grocery store. The golden-yellow powder can stain countertops and clothing, so handle it carefully. When stored in an airtight container, it will stay fresh for months.

Vanilla
Vanilla extract is a flavoring that many of us have in our spice cabinets. It adds a lot of flavor without adding many calories to smoothies. Look for vanilla that does not contain sugar; I recommend the Simply Organic brand. Whole vanilla beans can also be added to smoothies for an intense burst of rich vanilla flavor. Vanilla is of interest as a potential anticancer food because vanilla beans contain piperonal and vanillin, which are cytotoxic compounds that have been found to inhibit cancer cells in laboratory studies.

Water
Proper hydration is critical to the healing process. Use tap water that has been purified through a solid carbon filter, or use glass-bottled, filtered water. Purified water can also be used to make ice cubes, and the tea used in smoothies.

Watermelon

Frozen watermelon provides a lush, frosty texture. Watermelon is rich in carotenoids and adds a sweet, distinctive flavor that pairs well with berries and other melons. To prepare watermelon for smoothies, remove the rind and cut the melon into large chunks. Choose seedless watermelon if you prefer an even texture (no seed bits) in your smoothies. Once the rind is removed, watermelon chunks can be frozen to keep them fresh.

Wild Blueberries

Wild blueberries are more flavorful and colorful, and contain higher antioxidant levels than cultivated blueberries. They are sold online and in the freezer department of most grocery stores. Keep them in airtight containers or food storage bags in the freezer and they will stay fresh for months.

Banana Smoothies

Fresh and frozen bananas provide tropical flavor, creamy texture, and anticancer nutrients to smoothies. In addition to potassium and vitamin B6, they also contain prebiotics including inulin, fructo-oligosaccharides, and other oligosaccharides that help feed the probiotics (healthy bacteria) in our digestive tracts.

Bananas also contain the anticancer phenolic compounds catechin, gallocatechin, and epicatechin, as well as the antioxidant dopamine. Dopamine not only reduces oxidation and inflammation, but it also supports mood and relaxation. Another surprising compound discovered in bananas is melatonin, which is the molecule that helps regulate sleep.

Additionally, the banana peel, which is also edible in organic bananas, has been found to be useful in the treatment of benign prostate hyperplasia.

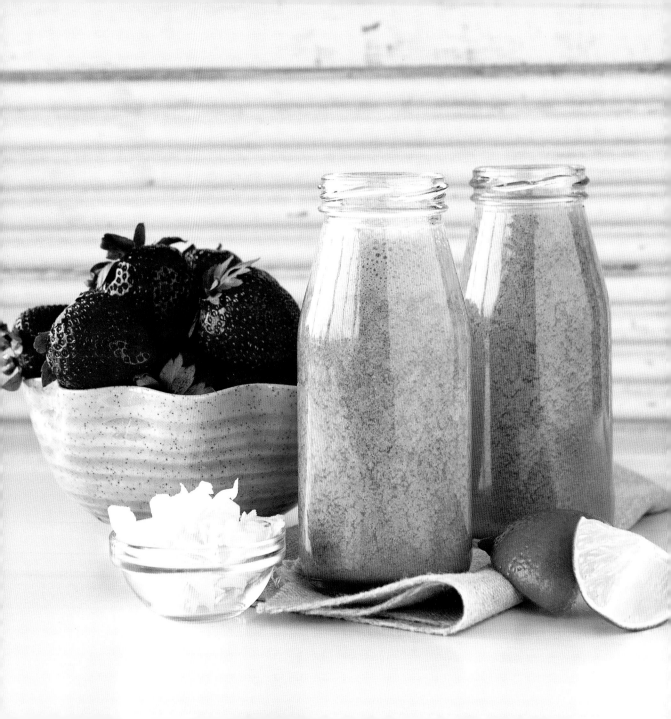

Tropical Lime

Bananas are an excellent source of antioxidants and prebiotics, which support the growth of the healthy bacteria in our digestive tracts.

This creamy banana and mango smoothie has a tea base, so it's not too sweet, and coconut gives this rich concoction the perfect balance of tropical flavors.

Ingredients

½ frozen banana
1 lime wedge
½ cup pomegranate juice
½ cup fresh mango
½ cup frozen green tea cubes
2 tablespoons shredded unsweetened coconut
2 tablespoons hulled hemp seed

Combine all ingredients in a high-power blender or food processor and blend until smooth. Drink immediately.

Serves: 2

Nutrition Facts (per serving)

Calories 228
Fat 12 g
Carbs 27 g
Fiber 5 g
Protein 4 g

Bennett RN, Shiga TM, Hassimotto NM, Rosa EA, Lajolo FM, Cordenunsi BR. (2010) Phenolics and antioxidant properties of fruit pulp and cell wall fractions of postharvest banana (Musa acuminata Juss.) cultivars. *Journal of Agricultural and Food Chemistry.*

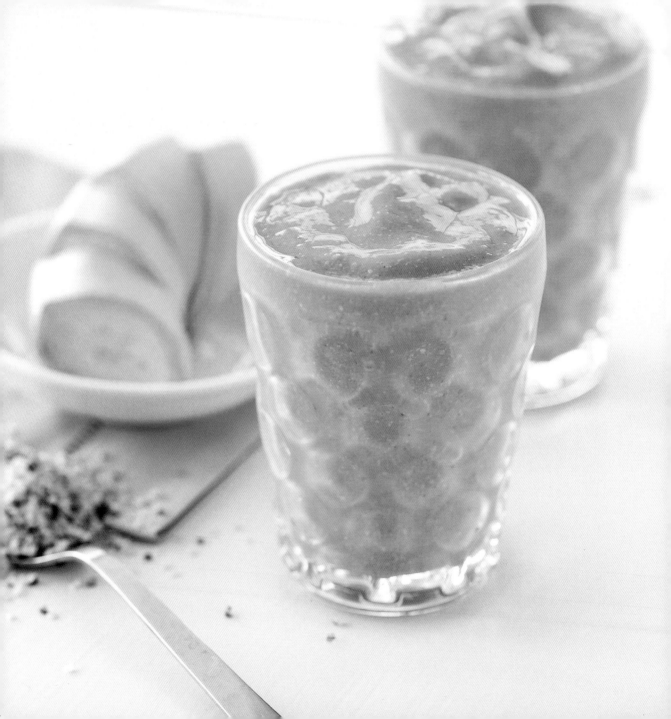

Mango Cream

Bananas are rich in dopamine, which means they can enhance our mood while the dopamine's antioxidant properties provide protection from cancer development.

This tropical blend has a smooth and creamy texture and subtle mango fragrance.

Ingredients

½ banana
½ cup carrot juice
½ cup frozen mango
½ cup frozen green tea
  cubes
2 tablespoons hulled
  hemp seed
1 teaspoon probiotic
  powder

Combine all ingredients in a high-power blender or food processor and blend until smooth. Drink immediately.

Serves 2

Nutrition Facts (per serving)

Calories 118
Fat 3 g
Carbs 20 g
Fiber 3 g
Protein 3 g

Kanazawa K, Sakakibara H. (2000) High content of dopamine, a strong antioxidant, in Cavendish banana. *Journal of Agricultural and Food Chemistry.*

Creamy Citrus Berry

Bananas contain phenolics such as catechin, gallocatechin, and epicatechin, which have remarkable antioxidant abilities that help protect us from cancer development and growth.

This lightly sweet blend is creamy, with subtle banana flavor, and is just slightly tart.

Ingredients

½ frozen banana
1 lime wedge
1 cup cultured coconut milk
½ cup blood orange
½ cup frozen strawberries
½ cup frozen green tea cubes
2 tablespoons protein powder

Combine all ingredients in a high-power blender or food processor and blend until smooth. Drink immediately.

Serves 2

Nutrition Facts (per serving)

Calories 96
Fat 1 g
Carbs 16 g
Fiber 4 g
Protein 7 g

Bennett RN, Shiga TM, Hassimotto NM, Rosa EA, Lajolo FM, Cordenunsi BR. (2010) Phenolics and antioxidant properties of fruit pulp and cell wall fractions of postharvest banana (Musa acuminata Juss.) cultivars. *Journal of Agricultural and Food Chemistry.*

Banana Ginger Dream

Researchers found that eating bananas increases body concentration of the sleep regulating molecule melatonin within two hours of consumption.

Creamy and sweet, this smoothie tastes like candied ginger with a little bit of fresh ginger heat.

Ingredients

½ frozen banana
½ cup orange juice
½ cup frozen peaches
½ cup frozen green tea
  cubes
2 tablespoons fresh ginger
  root
2 tablespoons protein
  powder

Combine all ingredients in a high-power blender or food processor and blend until smooth. Drink immediately.

Serves 2

Nutrition Facts (per serving)

Calories 93
Fat 0 g
Carbs 16 g
Fiber 1 g
Protein 7 g

Sae-Teaw M, Johns J, Johns NP, Subongkot S. (2012) Serum melatonin levels and antioxidant capacities after consumption of pineapple, orange, or banana by healthy male volunteers. *Journal of Pineal Research.*

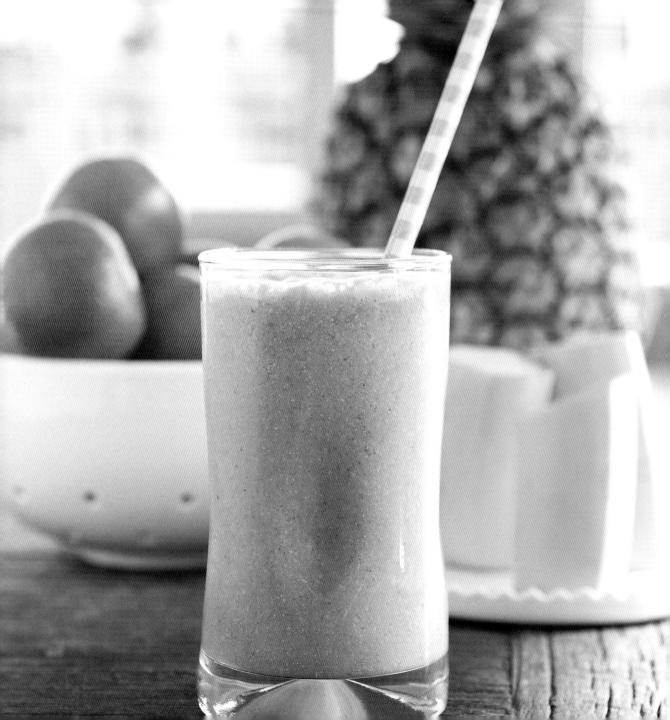

Sweet Citrus Carrot

Bananas contain prebiotics including inulin and fructo-oligosaccharides that stimulate the growth of beneficial gut flora such as Bifidobacterium, which not only improves digestion but also provides protection from fungal and bacterial infections.

This tropical blend is fresh and light with subtle sweet carrot flavor.

Ingredients

2 mandarin oranges
½ banana
½ cup pineapple
½ cup carrot juice
½ cup frozen green tea
   cubes
2 tablespoons hulled
   hemp seed

Combine all ingredients in a high-power blender or food processor and blend until smooth. Drink immediately.

Serves 2

Nutrition Facts (per serving)

Calories 168
Fat 3 g
Carbs 31 g
Fiber 3 g
Protein 4 g

Slavin J. (2013) Fiber and prebiotics: mechanisms and health benefits. *Nutrients Journal.*

Vanilla Bean Banana

Melatonin is a molecule that our bodies produce to help regulate our sleep cycles. However, it also provides protection against some neurodegenerative diseases and cancers. Researchers have found that pineapple, oranges, and banana are rich sources of this cancer protective molecule.

Light and creamy, this smoothie has subtle banana and vanilla flavors.

Ingredients

1 vanilla bean
½ frozen banana
½ cup orange juice
½ cup fresh pineapple
½ cup frozen green tea cubes
2 tablespoons protein powder

Combine all ingredients in a high-power blender or food processor and blend until smooth. Drink immediately.

Serves 2

Nutrition Facts (per serving)

Calories 107
Fat 0 g
Carbs 20 g
Fiber 2 g
Protein 7 g

Sae-Teaw M, Johns J, Johns NP, Subongkot S. (2012) Serum melatonin levels and antioxidant capacities after consumption of pineapple, orange, or banana by healthy male volunteers. *Journal of Pineal Research.*

Peanut Butter and Jelly

Resveratrol, which is found in red grapes and peanuts, reduces cancer growth and development by reducing inflammation.

This sweet and nutty smoothie tastes a lot like a peanut butter and jelly sandwich.

Ingredients

½ frozen banana
1 cup black currant juice
½ cup frozen green tea cubes
2 tablespoons peanut butter
2 tablespoons hulled hemp seed

Combine all ingredients in a high-power blender or food processor and blend until smooth. Drink immediately.

Serves 2

Nutrition Facts (per serving)

Calories 161
Fat 11 g
Carbs 10 g
Fiber 3 g
Protein 7 g

Khuda-Bukhsh AR, Das S, Saha SK. (2014) Molecular approaches toward targeted cancer prevention with some food plants and their products: inflammatory and other signal pathways. *Nutrition and Cancer.*

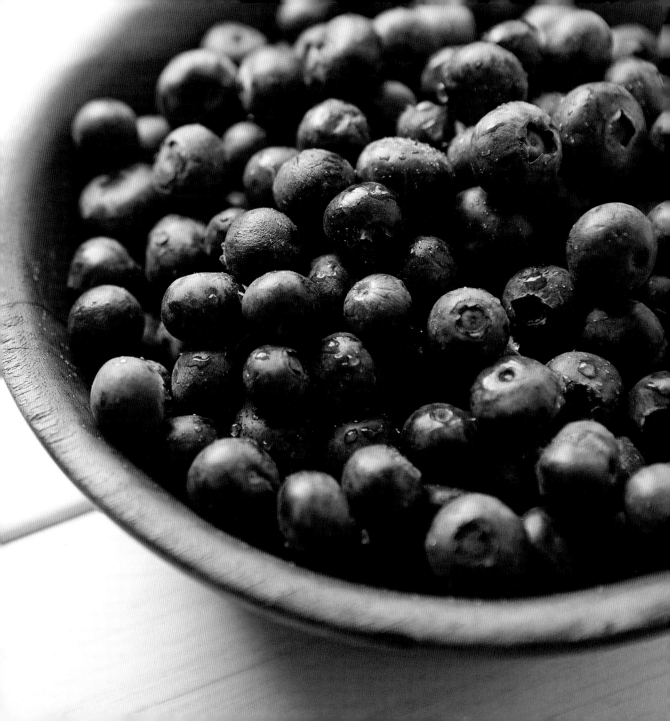

Berry Blends

Berries, berry juice, and berry juice concentrates are excellent smoothie ingredients. For example, blackberries, blueberries, cherries, cranberries, raspberries, and strawberries all provide rich, sweet flavor, as well as color, fragrance, and well-studied anticancer nutrients.

All berries contain "berry bioactives" and each berry contains specific compounds that act in their own way to reduce cancer in our bodies. For example, most berries contain flavonoids, proanthocyanidins, ellagitannins, gallotannins, phenolic acids, stilbenoids, lignans, and triterpenoids. However, strawberries in particular contain the flavonoid fisetin, while grapes contain resveratrol and phenols, and tart cherries are rich in anthocyanins, which support the inhibition of cancer cell growth.

Studies show that berry bioactives have anticancer properties such as their ability to counteract, reduce, and repair damage resulting from oxidative stress and inflammation. They also regulate toxin-metabolizing enzymes, various growth factors, inflammatory cytokines, and signaling pathways of cancer cell proliferation, apoptosis, and tumor angiogenesis.

These studies have found that berry nutrients affect specific types of cancer. For example, black raspberries are rich in polyphenolic anthocyanins, which have been shown to inhibit the development of esophageal cancer by influencing the genes associated with inflammation. Black raspberries also suppress ulcerative colitis by regulating inflammation.

Berries not only support healing; they also contain natural phytochemicals that enhance chemotherapy by reducing treatment resistance and providing protection from therapy-associated toxicities.

Researchers have also found that we can increase the absorption of these anticancer nutrients by ingesting probiotics, which are the healthy bacteria we need in our intestines to help us metabolize berry nutrients such as anthocyanins.

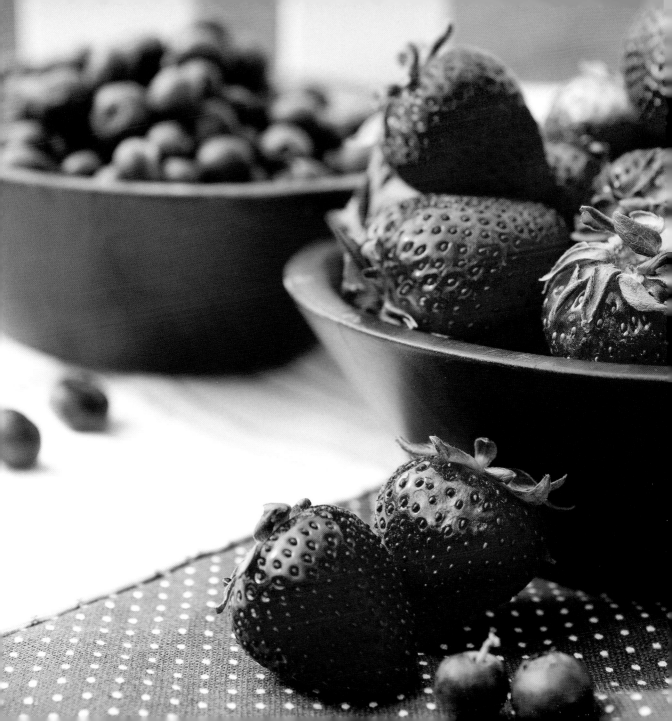

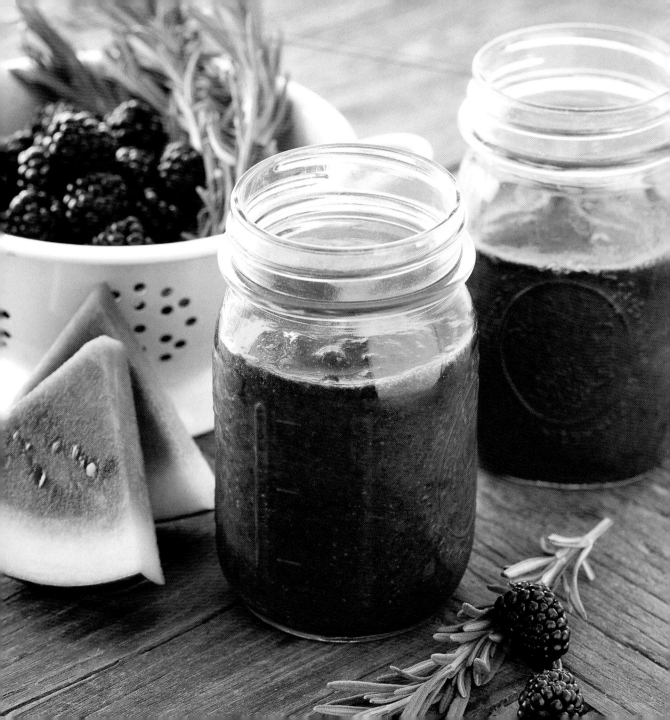

Watermelon Blackberry Citrus

Berries and berry juices contain active compounds that counteract, reduce, and repair damage to cells resulting from oxidative stress and inflammation.

The sweetness of the berries and the watermelon in this blend are balanced by the bitterness of the rosemary and the acidity of the lime. The bitter compounds in the rosemary support digestion and help stimulate the release of digestive enzymes and hydrochloric acid.

Ingredients

½ cup watermelon
½ cup coconut water
½ cup frozen blackberries
½ cup frozen green tea
    cubes
2 tablespoons lime juice
2 tablespoons hulled
    hemp seed
1 tablespoon fresh
    rosemary

Combine all ingredients in a high-power blender or food processor and blend until smooth. Drink immediately.

Serves 1

Nutrition Facts (per serving)

Calories 87
Fat 3 g
Carbs 12 g
Fiber 4 g
Protein 4 g

Seeram, NP. (2006) Blackberry, black raspberry, blueberry, cranberry, red raspberry, and strawberry extracts inhibit growth and stimulate apoptosis of human cancer cells in vitro. *Journal of Agricultural and Food Chemistry.*

Berry Carrot Ginger

Berries contain natural phytochemicals that support chemotherapy by reducing treatment resistance. Berry nutrients also provide protection from therapy-associated toxicities.

This complex smoothie has a fresh berry flavor and a creamy banana base with a little ginger bite.

Ingredients

½ banana
½ cup carrot juice
½ cup red raspberries
½ cup frozen green tea cubes
2 tablespoons fresh ginger root
2 tablespoons hulled hemp seed
½ teaspoon turmeric powder

Combine all ingredients in a high-power blender or food processor and blend until smooth. Drink immediately.

Serves 2

Nutrition Facts (per serving)

Calories 143
Fat 3 g
Carbs 26 g
Fiber 4 g
Protein 4 g

Seeram, NP. (2006) Blackberry, black raspberry, blueberry, cranberry, red raspberry, and strawberry extracts inhibit growth and stimulate apoptosis of human cancer cells in vitro. *Journal of Agricultural and Food Chemistry.*

Watermelon Cherry Rosemary

Tart cherries and tart cherry juice contain nutrients that improve antioxidant defenses, which provide cancer protection by reducing oxidative damage to nucleic acids.

This smoothie has a fresh pineapple flavor and a light rosemary fragrance.

Ingredients

½ cup watermelon
½ cup pineapple
½ cup frozen tart cherries
½ cup frozen green tea cubes
2 tablespoons chia seed
1 tablespoon fresh rosemary

Combine all ingredients in a high-power blender or food processor and blend until smooth. Drink immediately.

Serves 2

Nutrition Facts (per serving)

Calories 133
Fat 5 g
Carbs 17 g
Fiber 8 g
Protein 4 g

Traustadóttir T, Davies SS, Stock AA, Su Y, Heward CB, Roberts LJ 2nd, Harman SM. (2009) Tart cherry juice decreases oxidative stress in healthy older men and women. *Journal of Nutrition.*

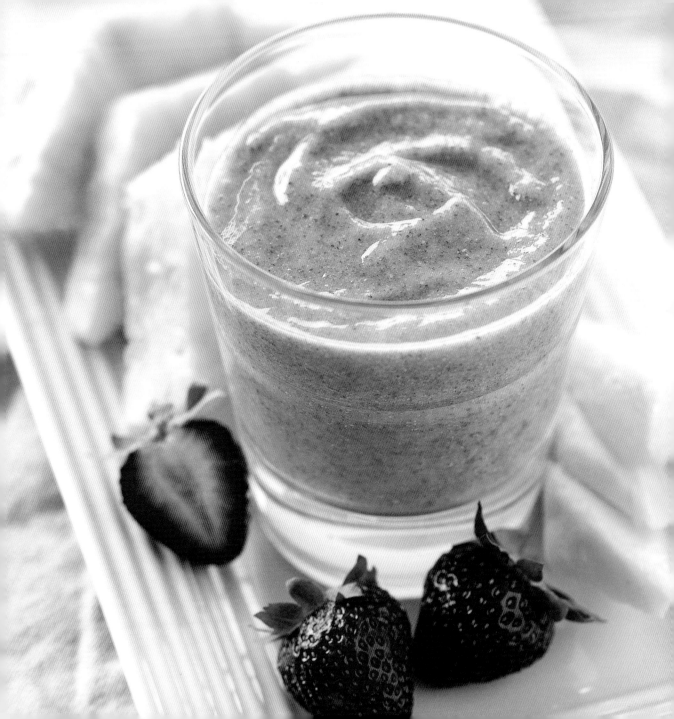

Berry Mango Citrus

Mango (the flesh and the skin) is a source of is a source of mangiferin, which is showing promise in inhibiting the growth of cancer.

This tropical medley is creamy and light with a pineapple fragrance.

Ingredients

½ cup coconut water
½ cup frozen strawberries
½ cup frozen mango
½ cup pineapple
½ tablespoon lemon juice
2 tablespoons chia seed

Combine all ingredients in a high-power blender or food processor and blend until smooth. Drink immediately.

Serves 2

Nutrition Facts (per serving)

Calories 144
Fat 5 g
Carbs 20 g
Fiber 8 g
Protein 4 g

Wilkinson AS, Flanagan BM, Pierson JT, Hewavitharana AK, Dietzgen RG, Shaw PN, Roberts-Thomson SJ, Monteith GR, Gidley MJ. (2011) Bioactivity of mango flesh and peel extracts on peroxisome proliferator-activated receptor γ [PPARγ] activation and MCF-7 cell proliferation: fraction and fruit variability. *Journal of Food Science*.

Watermelon Raspberry Cooler

Watermelon is rich in carotenoids, which reduce the risk of lung cancer development.

Tart and sweet, this watermelon and raspberry combination is balanced by tangy cranberry juice.

Ingredients

1 cup frozen green tea cubes
½ cup frozen red raspberries
½ cup watermelon
¼ cup cranberry juice
2 tablespoons chia seed

Combine all ingredients in a high-power blender or food processor and blend until smooth. Drink immediately.

Serves 2

Nutrition Facts (per serving)

Calories 160
Fat 4 g
Carbs 29 g
Fiber 8 g
Protein 3 g

Takata Y, Xiang YB, Yang G, Li H, Gao J, Cai H, Gao YT, Zheng W, Shu XO. (2013) Intakes of fruits, vegetables, and related vitamins and lung cancer risk: results from the Shanghai Men's Health Study (2002-2009). *Nutrition and Cancer.*

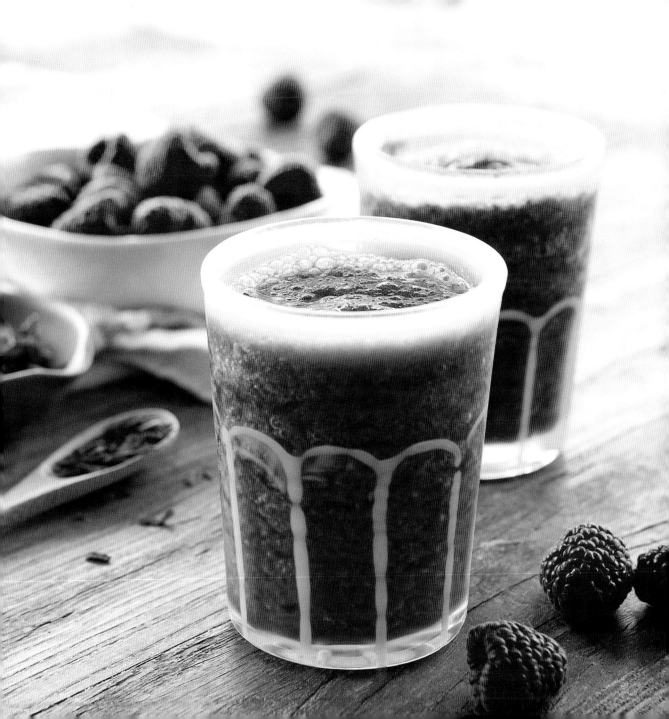

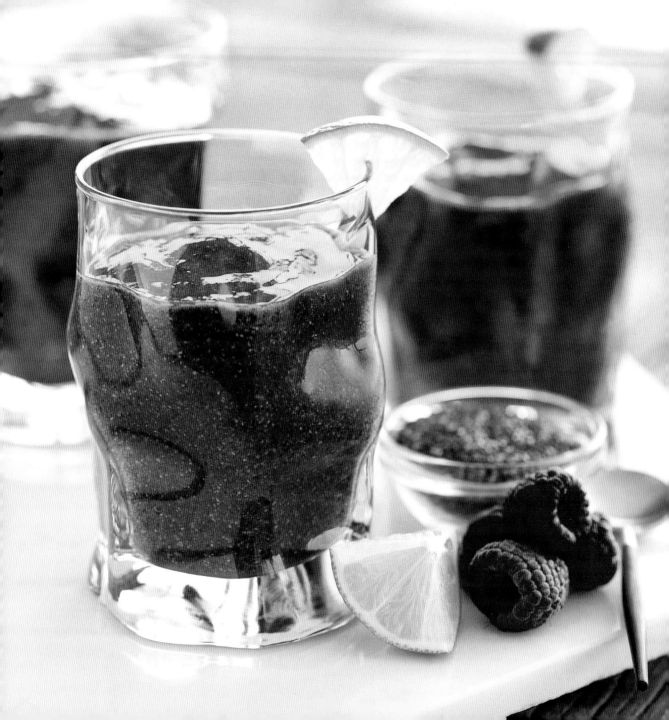

Cherry Berry Lime

Berries contain bioactive phytochemicals with anticancer actions such as apoptosis and inhibition of cancer development.

This tart and citrusy smoothie has a hint of sweetness and rich berry flavor.

Ingredients

¼ lime
½ cup tart cherry juice
½ cup frozen red
    raspberries
½ cup frozen green tea
    cubes
2 tablespoons chia seed

Combine all ingredients in a high-power blender or food processor and blend until smooth. Drink immediately.

Serves 2

Nutrition Facts (per serving)

Calories 161
Fat 5 g
Carbs 24 g
Fiber 9 g
Protein 4 g

Seeram, NP. (2006) Blackberry, black raspberry, blueberry, cranberry, red raspberry, and strawberry extracts inhibit growth and stimulate apoptosis of human cancer cells in vitro. *Journal of Agricultural and Food Chemistry.*

Kumquat Berry Cherry

Cranberries and cranberry juice have been shown to reduce growth of cancer cells via their anti-oxidative and anti-inflammatory properties.

This tart and intense smoothie has a cranberry and citrus base with a bit of sweet berry flavor.

Ingredients

2 kumquats
½ cup tart cherry juice
½ cup frozen strawberries
½ cup frozen green tea cubes
¼ cup cranberry juice
2 tablespoons chia seed
1 tablespoon fresh rosemary

Combine all ingredients in a high-power blender or food processor and blend until smooth. Drink immediately.

Serves 2

Nutrition Facts (per serving)

Calories 129
Fat 5 g
Carbs 16 g
Fiber 7 g
Protein 4 g

Katsargyris A, Tampaki EC, Giaginis C, Theocharis S. (2012) Cranberry as promising natural source of potential anticancer agents: current evidence and future perspectives. *Anticancer Agents in Medicinal Chemistry*.

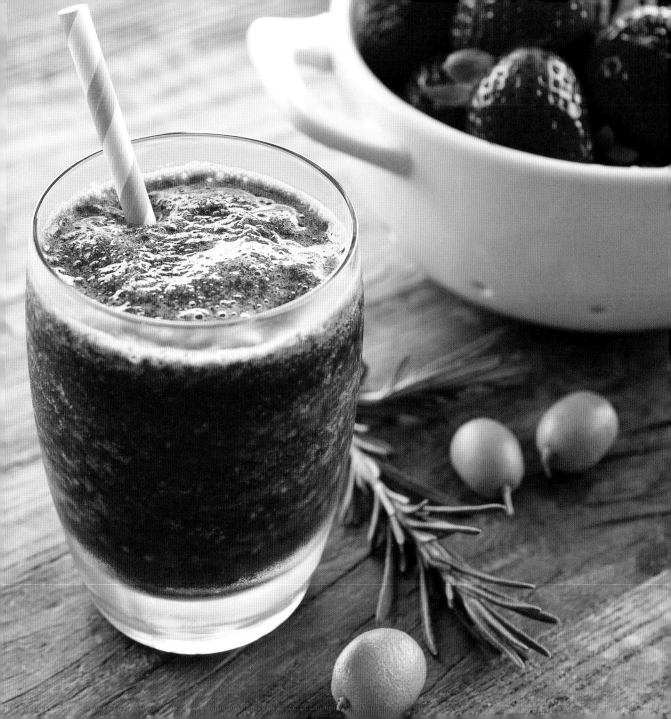

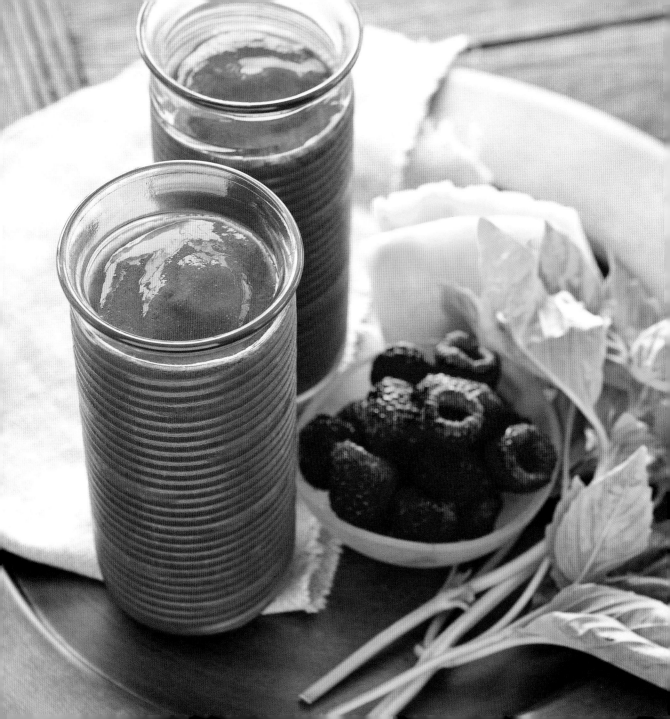

Basil Pom Pine

The core of the pineapple is a rich source of bromelain, a proteolytic enzyme, which has been found to reduce the growth and spread of gastrointestinal cancers. This anticancer enzyme also provides protection from development of new cancer cells and has been reported to promote apoptosis in many types of cancer.

Basil and melon complement each other in this fruity blend.

Ingredients

½ cup fresh basil leaves
½ cup pomegranate juice
½ cup frozen pineapple
½ cup watermelon
½ cup frozen red
  raspberries
½ cup frozen green tea
  cubes
2 tablespoons chia seed

Combine all ingredients in a high-power blender or food processor and blend until smooth. Drink immediately.

Serves 2

Nutrition Facts (per serving)

Calories 209
Fat 5 g
Carbs 36 g
Fiber 10 g
Protein 4 g

Romano B, Fasolino I, Pagano E, Capasso R, Pace S, De Rosa G, Milic N, Orlando P, Izzo AA, Borrelli F. (2014) The chemopreventive action of bromelain, from pineapple stem (Ananas comosus L.), on colon carcinogenesis is related to antiproliferative and proapoptotic effects. *Molecular Nutrition & Food Research.*

Cherry Coconut

Tart cherries are rich in anthocyanins, which have been found to protect against colon cancer.

Rich cherry flavor with a little coconut fragrance, this smoothie is simple and rich in protein.

Ingredients

½ cup coconut water
½ cup frozen tart cherries
½ cup frozen green tea
  cubes
2 tablespoons protein
  powder

Combine all ingredients in a high-power blender or food processor and blend until smooth. Drink immediately.

Serves 1

Nutrition Facts (per serving)

Calories 93
Fat 0 g
Carbs 9 g
Fiber 1 g
Protein 13 g

Kang SY, Seeram NP, Nair MG, Bourquin LD. (2003) Tart cherry anthocyanins inhibit tumor development in Apc(Min) mice and reduce proliferation of human colon cancer cells. *Cancer Letters.*

Berry Citrus Cream

Strawberries contain anti-inflammatory phenolics that can be absorbed by our intestines when metabolized by probiotics such as those in cultured coconut milk.

This thick and rich strawberry smoothie is sweet and creamy with a heady vanilla fragrance and notes of tart citrus.

Ingredients

½ cup vanilla flavored
   cultured coconut milk
½ cup orange juice
½ cup frozen strawberries
½ cup frozen green tea
   cubes
2 tablespoons chia seed

Combine all ingredients in a high-power blender or food processor and blend until smooth. Drink immediately.

Serves 1

Nutrition Facts (per serving)

Calories 241
Fat 13 g
Carb 22 g
Fiber 14 g
Protein 7 g

Giampieri F, Alvarez-Suarez JM, Battino M. (2014) Strawberry and Human Health: Effects beyond Antioxidant Activity. *Journal of Agricultural and Food Chemistry.*

Tarko T, Duda-Chodak A, Zajac N. (2013) Digestion and absorption of phenolic compounds assessed by in vitro simulation methods. *Annals of the National Institute of Hygiene.*

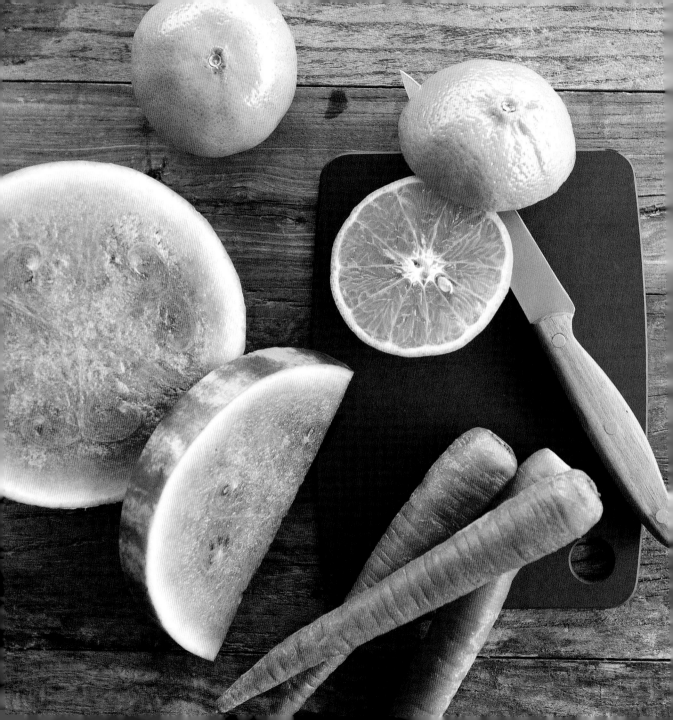

Carotenoid Boosters

Carotenoids including alpha- and beta-carotene are nutrients found in fruit like apricots, carrots, cherries, cantaloupe, mangos, peaches, plums, strawberries, tangerines, and watermelon.

These nutrients are rich in color so we see them in our produce as colors ranging from pale yellow to deep red.

We have long known that people who eat a diet rich in fruits and vegetables have higher blood levels of these nutrients and lower incidence of diseases including cancer.

Researchers are now finding that these compounds act in very specific ways to reduce cancer. For example, they act as antioxidants reducing oxidative stress and inflammation. They also enhance detoxification processes in our bodies, reducing the toxic burden that can lead to cancer development.

Basil Berry Citrus

Basil and turmeric are a powerful ovarian-cancer fighting team. Curcumin, which is the bioactive compound in turmeric, significantly enhances the ability of basil polysaccharides to decrease the invasion activity of ovarian cancer cells.

This berry and citrus smoothie has a subtle tea flavor and basil fragrance.

Ingredients

½ cup orange juice
½ cup frozen raspberries
½ cup frozen green tea
   cubes
½ cup fresh basil leaves
2 tablespoons chia seed
¼ teaspoon turmeric
   powder

Combine all ingredients in a high-power blender or food processor and blend until smooth. Drink immediately.

Serves 1

Nutrition Facts (per serving)

Calories 156
Fat 5 g
Carbs 22 g
Fiber 9 g
Protein 4 g

Lv J, Shao Q, Wang H, Shi H, Wang T, Gao W, Song B, Zheng G, Kong B, Qu X. (2013) Effects and mechanisms of curcumin and basil polysaccharide on the invasion of SKOV3 cells and dendritic cells. *Molecular Medicine Reports.*

Cherry Carrot

Daily intake of fresh carrot juice increases the carotenoids in the blood, which reduces oxidative stress and has been found to provide protection from recurrence in women previously treated for breast cancer.

This earthy and wholesome smoothie has a fresh scent and a subtle sweet flavor that makes it one of those perfect "daily" smoothies.

Ingredients

½ cup carrot juice
½ cup frozen pineapple
½ cup frozen dark sweet
  cherries
½ cup frozen green tea
  cubes
2 tablespoons hulled
  hemp seed

Combine all ingredients in a high-power blender or food processor and blend until smooth. Drink immediately.

Serves 2

Nutrition Facts (per serving)

Calories 108
Fat 3 g
Carbs 17 g
Fiber 3 g
Protein 3 g

Butalla AC, Crane TE, Patil B, Wertheim BC, Thompson P, Thomson CA. (2012) Effects of a carrot juice intervention on plasma carotenoids, oxidative stress, and inflammation in overweight breast cancer survivors. *Nutrition and Cancer.*

Carotenoid Crush

Pineapple contains bromelain, which not only helps prevent colon cancer but also reduces growth of existing colon cancer and triggers apoptosis.

Bromelain, which is a mixture of enzymes derived from pineapple, decreases the inflammation associated with colon cancer. Fresh, frozen, and unpasteurized pineapple juice all contain bromelain.

This fragrant fruity combination has a tropical flavor with a light citrus finish.

Ingredients

½ cup orange juice
½ cup frozen peaches
½ cup frozen strawberries
½ cup pineapple
½ cup frozen green tea
  cubes
2 tablespoons protein
  powder

Combine all ingredients in a high-power blender or food processor and blend until smooth. Drink immediately.

Serves 2

Nutrition Facts (per serving)

Calories 112
Fat 0 g
Carbs 21 g
Fiber 2 g
Protein 7g

Romano B, Fasolino I, Pagano E, Capasso R, Pace S, De Rosa G, Milic N, Orlando P, Izzo AA, Borrelli F. (2014) The chemopreventive action of bromelain, from pineapple stem (Ananas comosus L.), on colon carcinogenesis is related to antiproliferative and proapoptotic effects. *Molecular Nutrition & Food Research.*

Hale LP, Chichlowski M, Trinh CT, Greer PK. (2010) Dietary supplementation with fresh pineapple juice decreases inflammation and colonic neoplasia in IL-10-deficient mice with colitis. *Inflammatory Bowel Disease.*

Blackberry Lemonade

One of the ways that probiotics reduce the incidence of colon cancer is by reducing inflammation. Probiotics can be added directly to smoothies in powder form.

This berry and citrus smoothie is like a red lemon candy with layers of fruit flavor.

Ingredients

1 cup green tea
½ cup fresh mango
½ cup frozen blackberries
½ cup frozen strawberries
2 tablespoons protein
   powder
1 tablespoon lemon juice
1 teaspoon probiotic
   powder

Combine all ingredients in a high-power blender or food processor and blend until smooth. Drink immediately.

Serves 2

Nutrition Facts (per serving)

Calories 99
Fat 0 g
Carbs 17 g
Fiber 5 g
Protein 8 g

Ewaschuk JB, Walker JW, Diaz H, Madsen KL. (2006) Bioproduction of conjugated linoleic acid by probiotic bacteria occurs in vitro and in vivo in mice. *Journal of Nutrition.*

Summer Thirst Quencher

Citrus pulp and juice contain cryptoxanthin, a carotenoid, as well as hesperidin, a flavonoid, which inhibit cancer by increasing the action of detoxifying enzymes and reducing inflammation.

Keep a glass bottle of unfiltered lemon juice in the refrigerator and add a tablespoon to each of your smoothies to get these benefits in your own blends.

This intensely flavorful and mouthwatering blend of healing fruit is energizing and hydrating.

Ingredients

½ cup watermelon
½ cup frozen strawberries
½ cup pomegranate juice
½ cup frozen green tea
  cubes
2 tablespoons chia seed
1 tablespoon lemon juice

Combine all ingredients in a high-power blender or food processor and blend until smooth. Drink immediately.

Serves 2

Nutrition Facts (per serving)

Calories 133
Fat 5 g
Carbs 17 g
Fiber 7 g
Protein 4 g

Tanaka T, Tanaka T, Tanaka M, Kuno T. (2011) Cancer chemoprevention by citrus pulp and juices containing high amounts of β-cryptoxanthin and hesperidin. *BioMed Research International.*

Berry Carrot Fresh

Healthy fats such as those in olive oil, chia seed, and hulled hemp seed significantly reduce the protein activities of lipogenic enzymes associated with cancer cell growth.

Adding a tablespoon of these fat-rich foods to your daily smoothie is an effective and safe way to reduce cancer cell growth.

This smoothie has fresh berry and carrot fragrance. The tart tang of tangerine and sweet strawberries is balanced by the tea and carrot.

Ingredients

½ cup carrot juice
½ cup strawberries
½ cup tangerine
½ cup frozen green tea cubes
2 tablespoons hulled hemp seed

Combine all ingredients in a high-power blender or food processor and blend until smooth. Drink immediately.

Serves 2

Nutrition Facts (per serving)

Calories 100
Fat 3 g
Carbs 15 g
Fiber 3 g
Protein 3 g

Notarnicola M, Tutino V, Caruso MG. (2014) Tumor-Induced Alterations in Lipid Metabolism. *Current Medicinal Chemistry.*

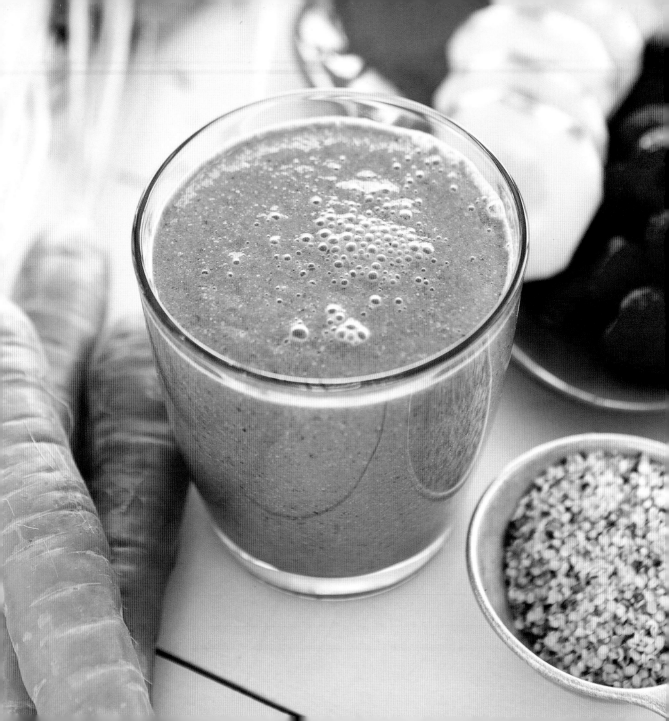

Carrot Currant Berry

Cucumbers contain anticancer compounds such as fisetin, lutein, and cucurbitacins, which inhibit prostate cancer growth.

This bright smoothie has a mouthwatering fragrance and is lightly sweet and tart with soft currant flavor.

Ingredients

¼ cup carrot juice
½ cup frozen raspberries
½ cup peeled cucumber
¼ cup currant juice
2 tablespoons hulled
 hemp seed

Combine all ingredients in a high-power blender or food processor and blend until smooth. Drink immediately.

Serves 2

Nutrition Facts (per serving)

Calories 118
Fat 3 g
Carbs 20 g
Fiber 4 g
Protein 3 g

Gao Y, Islam MS, Tian J, Lui VW, Xiao D. (2014) Inactivation of ATP citrate lyase by Cucurbitacin B: A bioactive compound from cucumber inhibits prostate cancer growth. *Cancer Letters*.

Grapefruit Rosemary

Nobiletin is one of the bioflavonoids found in citrus fruits such as lemons, oranges, tangerines, and grapefruits. Nobiletin has anti-inflammatory and anticancer actions and the potential to suppress metastasis of breast cancer.

This frosty blend has a perfect balance of citrus with a hint of bitterness from the grapefruit and rosemary. The flavor and fragrance are energizing, making this an excellent morning blend.

Ingredients

1 cup grapefruit
½ cup cherries
½ cup orange juice
½ cup frozen green tea cubes
2 tablespoons hulled hemp seed
1 tablespoon fresh rosemary

Combine all ingredients in a high-power blender or food processor and blend until smooth. Drink immediately.

Serves 2

Nutrition Facts (per serving)

Calories 144
Fat 3 g
Carbs 25 g
Fiber 2 g
Protein 4 g

Baek SH, Kim SM, Nam D, Lee JH, Ahn KS, Choi SH, Kim SH, Shim BS, Chang IM, Ahn KS. (2012) Antimetastatic effect of nobiletin through the down-regulation of CXC chemokine receptor type 4 and matrix metallopeptidase-9. *Pharmaceutical Biology.*

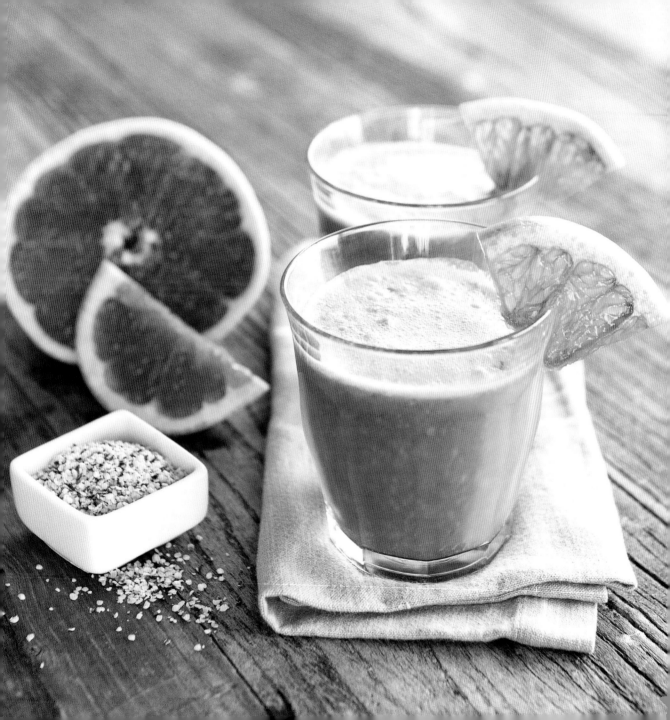

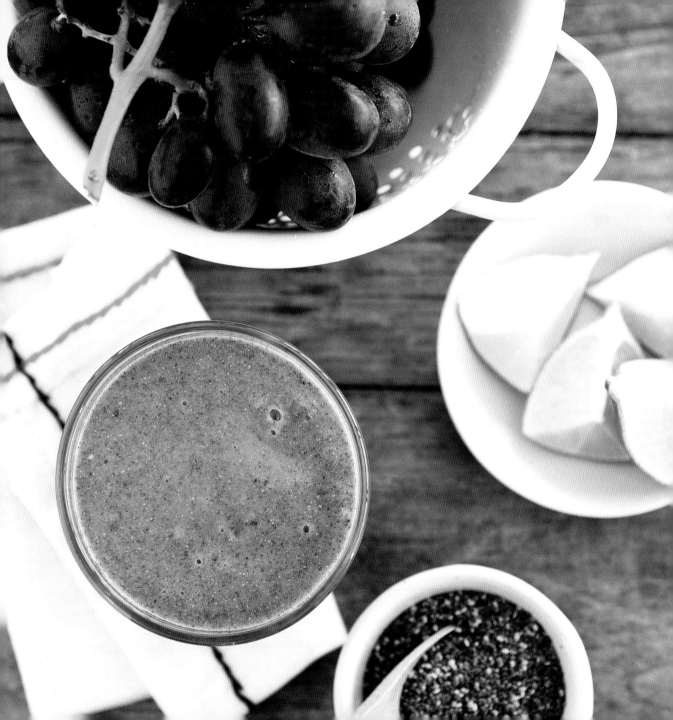

Currant Grape Tea

Berries provide quercetin, which is a flavonoid known for its ability to reduce the severity of allergic reactions and reduce cancer-induced inflammation.

This intense, fruity combination has a light tea and citrus fragrance.

Ingredients

1 lime wedge
½ cup currant juice
½ cup frozen grapes
½ cup watermelon
½ cup frozen green tea
 cubes
2 tablespoons chia seed

Combine all ingredients in a high-power blender or food processor and blend until smooth. Drink immediately.

Serves 2

Nutrition Facts (per serving)

Calories 127
Fat 5 g
Carbs 16 g
Fiber 7 g
Protein 4 g

Erlund I, Freese R, Marniemi J, Hakala P, Alfthan G. (2006) Bioavailability of quercetin from berries and the diet. *Nutrition and Cancer.*

Carotenoid Blend

Vitamin C in citrus fruits, carotenoids in carrots, and the myrecitin in cranberry juice affect signaling pathways that direct apoptosis and may be important factors in the treatment of cancer.

The number of ingredients in this recipe makes it a bit daunting to blend up frequently. However, it is the perfect smoothie to make into frozen smoothie cubes to have on hand for busy days. Just add a couple of frozen Carotenoid Blend smoothie cubes to a glass of water or juice for a rich dose of nutrients each day.

This light-peach colored, creamy smoothie has a fresh fragrance and is full of carotenoids from the watermelon as well as the cranberry and carrot juices.

Ingredients

¼ cup orange juice
¼ cup watermelon
¼ cup cranberry juice
¼ cup carrot juice
¼ cup frozen mango
¼ cup frozen green tea cubes
2 tablespoons hulled hemp seed
1 tablespoon lemon juice

Combine all ingredients in a high-power blender or food processor and blend until smooth. Drink immediately.

Serves 2

Nutrition Facts (per serving)

Calories 98
Fat 3 g
Carbs 15 g
Fiber 2 g
Protein 3 g

Khuda-Bukhsh AR, Das S, Saha SK. (2014) Molecular approaches toward targeted cancer prevention with some food plants and their products: inflammatory and other signal pathways. *Nutrition and Cancer.*

Citrus Blends

Ingesting citrus fruits, their juices, and even their peels on a regular basis, has been found to support cancer recovery in specific ways. Citrus fruits including oranges, grapefruit, kumquat, lemon, lime, and tangerines not only provide immune-supporting vitamin C but also specific anticancer compounds such as nobiletin, naringin, tangeretin, β-cryptoxanthin, and hesperidin. Naringin, for example, is a flavanone in citrus fruits, which acts as an antioxidant that reduces inflammation and has been found to provide protection against oral, breast, colon, liver, lung, and ovarian cancers.

Each citrus fruit contains its own group of active anticancer compounds; for example, blood orange contains carotenoids, ascorbic acid, hydroxycinnamic acids, and anthocyanins, while grapefruit contains nobiletin and lycopene, and lemons contain tangeretin and limonoids. Kumquats contain lutein, zeaxanthin, and tannins.

Current research has found that citrus peel oils contain concentrations of many of the bioactives found in the fruit. This definitely warrants adding some of the nutrient-rich citrus peel to smoothies.

Key Lime Swirl

Cow's milk contains hormones that increase prostate cancer growth. In fourteen separate experiments, researchers found that ingesting cow's milk increased prostate cancer cell growth at a rate of more than 30 percent. In contrast, almond milk suppressed the growth of these cells by more than 30 percent.

The lime peel essence really pops in this creamy rich smoothie.

Ingredients

½ lime with peel
½ cup almond milk
½ cup cultured coconut milk
½ cup frozen green tea cubes
2 tablespoons chia seed

Combine all ingredients in a high-power blender or food processor and blend until smooth. Drink immediately.

Serves 1

Nutrition Facts (per serving)

Calories 195
Fat 13 g
Carbs 9 g
Fiber 15 g
Protein 7 g

Tate PL, Bibb R, Larcom LL. (2011) Milk stimulates growth of prostate cancer cells in culture. *Nutrition and Cancer.*

Kumquat Cherry Citrus

Cherries, cherry juice, and cherry concentrates are all rich sources of polyphenol anthocyanins that contribute to the process of apoptosis, the destruction of cancer cells.

This tart and sweet blend has bright cherry and citrus flavor and fragrance.

Ingredients

2 kumquats
½ cup orange juice
½ cup cherries
½ cup frozen green tea cubes
2 tablespoons chia seed

Combine all ingredients in a high-power blender or food processor and blend until smooth. Drink immediately.

Serves 1

Nutrition Facts (per serving)

Calories 243
Fat 10 g
Carbs 27 g
Fiber 14 g
Protein 8 g

Martin KR, Wooden A. (2012) Tart Cherry Juice Induces Differential Dose-Dependent Effects on Apoptosis, But Not Cellular Proliferation, in MCF-7 Human Breast Cancer Cells. *Journal of Medicinal Food.*

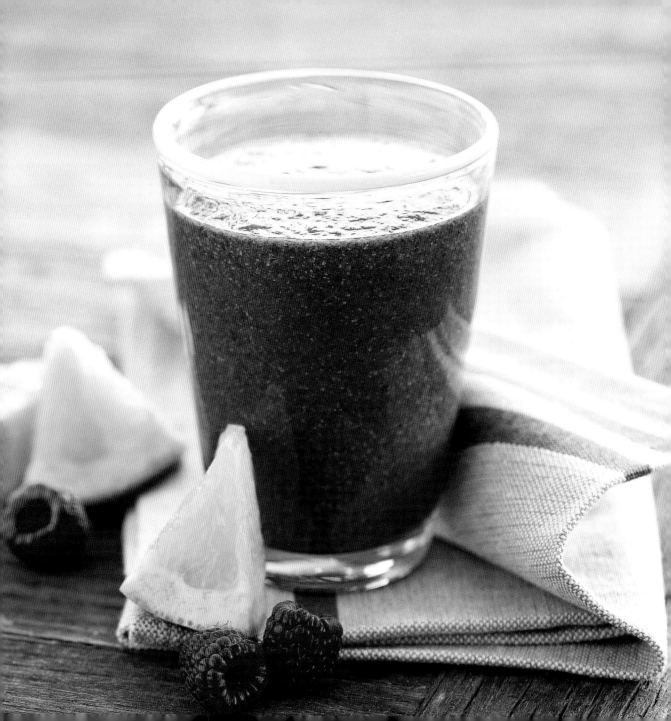

Melon Berry Citrus

Naringenin is a flavonoid, found in grapefruit and oranges, that acts as an antioxidant to provide protection from genetic mutations that can lead to cancer.

This blend is cool, lush and slightly tart with rich fruit flavor.

Ingredients

½ cup grapefruit
½ cup watermelon
½ cup frozen red
  raspberries
½ cup pomegranate juice
½ cup frozen green tea
  cubes
2 tablespoons chia seed

Combine all ingredients in a high-power blender or food processor and blend until smooth. Drink immediately.

Serves 2

Nutrition Facts (per serving)

Calories 194
Fat 5 g
Carbs 38 g
Fiber 8 g
Protein 4 g

Charles C, Nachtergael A, Ouedraogo M, Belayew A, Duez P. (2014) Effects of chemopreventive natural products on non-homologous end-joining DNA double-strand break repair. *Mutation Research*.

Citrus Cherry Mango

Cherries are anticarcinogenic because they are low-glycemic, anti-inflammatory, and rich in anthocyanins, quercetin, potassium, fiber, vitamin C, carotenoids, and melatonin.

This fresh blend is creamy with layers of subtle fruit flavor.

Ingredients

2 mandarin oranges
½ cup orange juice
½ cup mango
½ cup cherries
½ cup frozen green tea
    cubes
2 tablespoons hulled
    hemp seed

Combine all ingredients in a high-power blender or food processor and blend until smooth. Drink immediately.

Serves 2

Nutrition Facts (per serving)

Calories 190
Fat 5 g
Carbs 37 g
Fiber 8 g
Protein 5 g

McCune LM, Kubota C, Stendell-Hollis NR, Thomson CA. (2011) Cherries and health: a review. *Critical Reviews in Food Science and Nutrition*.

Watermelon Berry Crush

Limonoids are the bitter parts of citrus seeds that exhibit a wide range of biological properties, including anticancer, antibacterial, antifungal, antimalarial, and antiviral activities.

This creamy, rich, and slightly sweet smoothie has fresh, light citrus flavor.

Ingredients

½ orange
½ cup watermelon
½ cup frozen red
   raspberries
½ cup green tea
2 tablespoons chia seed

Combine all ingredients in a high-power blender or food processor and blend until smooth. Drink immediately.

Serves 1

Nutrition Facts (per serving)

Calories 169
Fat 5 g
Carbs 27 g
Fiber 11 g
Protein 4 g

Tundis R, Loizzo MR, Menichini F. (2014) An overview on chemical aspects and potential health benefits of limonoids and their derivatives. *Critical Reviews in Food Science and Nutrition.*

Fruit Punch Smoothie

Resveratrol is a naturally derived phytoalexin stilbene found in grapes and other plants that is well known for its properties as an antioxidant, anti–inflammatory, and anticancer agent.

This grapefruit smoothie is sweet and bitter and deliciously mouthwatering.

Ingredients

½ cup frozen grapes
½ cup orange juice
½ cup pineapple
½ cup grapefruit
½ cup frozen green tea
  cubes
2 tablespoons hulled
  hemp seed

Combine all ingredients in a high-power blender or food processor and blend until smooth. Drink immediately.

Serves 2

Nutrition Facts (per serving)

Calories 179
Fat 5 g
Carbs 35 g
Fiber 6 g
Protein 4 g

Xue YQ, Di JM, Luo Y, Cheng KJ, Wei X, Shi Z. (2014) Resveratrol Oligomers for the Prevention and Treatment of Cancers. *Oxidative Medicine Cellular Longevity Journal*.

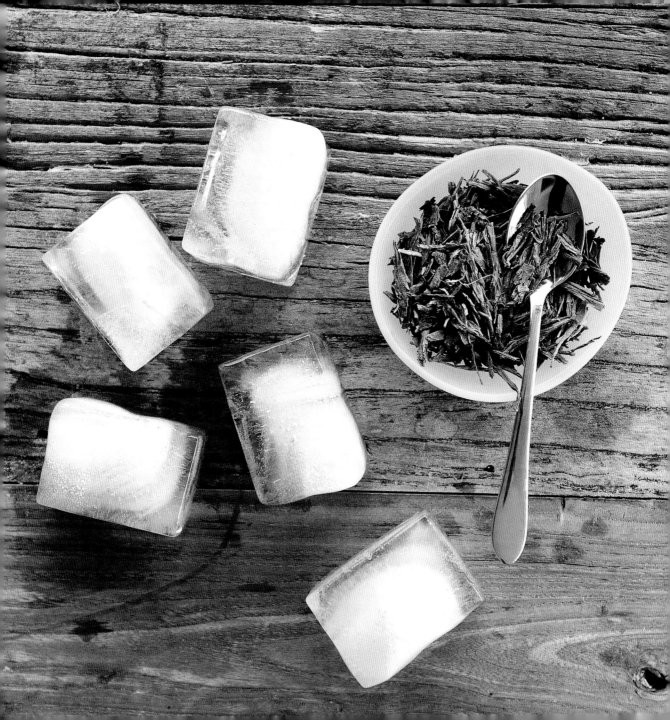

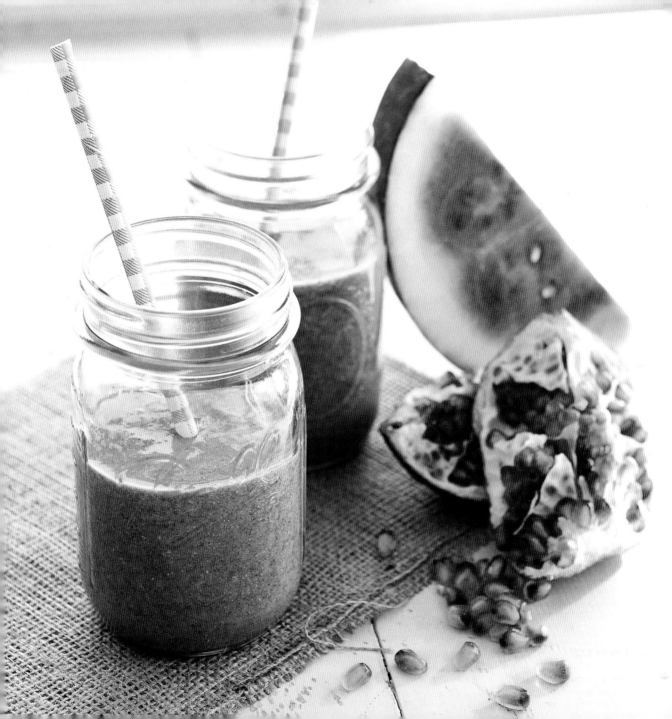

Pomegranate Punch

Lycopene is a carotenoid found in watermelon, pink grapefruit, tomato, and guava in high concentration. Dietary intake of lycopene provides protection against cellular damage that can lead to cancer development and growth.

This rich and frosty smoothie has a heady citrus scent and the flavors of summer.

Ingredients

½ cup fresh watermelon
½ cup orange juice
½ cup pomegranate seeds
½ cup frozen green tea
   cubes
2 tablespoons chia seed

Combine all ingredients in a high-power blender or food processor and blend until smooth. Drink immediately.

Serves 2

Nutrition Facts (per serving)

Calories 151
Fat 5 g
Carbs 20 g
Fiber 8 g
Protein 5 g

Agca CA, Tuzcu M, Gencoglu H, Akdemir F, Ali S, Sahin K, Kucuk O. (2012) Lycopene counteracts the hepatic response to 7,12-dimethylbenz[a]anthracene by altering the expression of Bax, Bcl-2, caspases, and oxidative stress biomarkers. *Pharmaceutical Biology.*

Crimson Candy

Pomegranate and pomegranate juice contain ellagic acid, which has been found to reduce hormone-sensitive breast cancer development.

This smoothie tastes tangy, like a sweet and sour candy, and has a bright candy color.

Ingredients

1 cup blood orange
½ cup pomegranate juice
½ cup frozen green tea cubes
½ cup frozen red raspberries
2 tablespoons chia seed

Combine all ingredients in a high-power blender or food processor and blend until smooth. Drink immediately.

Serves 2

Nutrition Facts (per serving)

Calories 205
Fat 5 g
Carbs 35 g
Fiber 11 g
Protein 4 g

Munagala R, Aqil F, Vadhanam MV, Gupta RC. (2013) MicroRNA 'signature' during estrogen-mediated mammary carcinogenesis and its reversal by ellagic acid intervention. *Cancer Letters*.

Kumquat Cherry

Limonoids, which are the bitter part of citrus seeds, provide a range of health benefits as they reduce bacterial, fungal, and viral infections. Their bitter flavor alone helps stimulate hydrochloric acid, which in turn helps dissolve infectious agents in the stomach.

This lush pink smoothie is rich and exotic with layers of tart, sweet, and citrus flavors.

Ingredients

2 kumquats
½ cup tart cherry juice
½ cup frozen strawberries
½ cup frozen green tea
 cubes
2 tablespoons chia seed

Combine all ingredients in a high-power blender or food processor and blend until smooth. Drink immediately.

Serves 2

Nutrition Facts (per serving)

Calories 114
Fat 5 g
Carbs 12 g
Fiber 7 g
Protein 4 g

Tundis R, Loizzo MR, Menichini F. (2014) An overview on chemical aspects and potential health benefits of limonoids and their derivatives. *Critical Reviews in Food Science and Nutrition.*

Tart Cherry Citrus

Saponins and phenolic compounds in tea inhibit the growth and spread of lymphoma cells.

This healthy blend tastes like candy and is sweet, fresh, and crisp.

Ingredients

¼ cup grapefruit
½ cup tart cherry juice
½ cup frozen strawberries
½ cup frozen white tea
   cubes
2 tablespoons chia seed

Combine all ingredients in a high-power blender or food processor and blend until smooth. Drink immediately.

Serves 1

Nutrition Facts (per serving)

Calories 253
Fat 10 g
Carbs 29 g
Fiber 14 g
Protein 8 g

Bhardwaj J, Chaudhary N, Seo HJ, Kim MY, Shin TS, Kim JD. (2014) Immunomodulatory effect of tea saponin in immune T-cells and T-lymphoma cells via regulation of Th1, Th2 immune response and MAPK/ERK2 signaling pathway. *Immunopharmacology and Immunotoxicology.*

Cocoa Dream Blends

Unsweetened cocoa powder and cocoa nibs are healthful additions that bring rich flavor and chocolate fragrance to smoothies.

Cocoa contains procyanidins, epicatechin, and catechins, which offer protection to our vascular and neurological systems. Cocoa contains theobromine as well, which protects against cancer, inflammation, and tumor development. Cocoa is also rich in the mineral magnesium, which increases relaxation, enhances sleep, and lowers blood pressure. Cocoa also contains flavonoids that have been found in numerous studies to reduce the growth and spread of cancer cells.

Cocoa Pom

Cocoa contains catechins that provide protection against stroke and other neurological damage. Cocoa is rich in procyanidins, theobromine, epicatechin, and catechins.

This rich, chocolate smoothie is a healthy alternative to a sweet dessert.

Ingredients

½ cup frozen banana
½ cup orange wedges
½ cup frozen green tea cubes
½ cup pomegranate juice
2 tablespoons unsweetened cocoa powder
2 tablespoons protein powder

Combine all ingredients in a high-power blender or food processor and blend until smooth. Drink immediately.

Serves 2

Nutrition Facts (per serving)

Calories 127
Fat 1 g
Carbs 22 g
Fiber 4 g
Protein 8 g

Kim J, Shim J, Lee CY, Lee KW, Lee HJ. (2014) Cocoa phytochemicals: recent advances in molecular mechanisms on health. *Critical Reviews in Food Science and Nutrition.*

Cocoa Light

Theobromine found in cocoa provides anti-tumor and anti-inflammatory effects.

This rich and creamy smoothie tastes like a chocolate milkshake but it's lower in calories, fat, and sugar and contains protein, fiber, and the cancer-reducing, natural plant compound theobromine.

Ingredients

½ cup frozen banana
½ cup coconut water
½ cup frozen green tea cubes
2 tablespoons unsweetened cocoa powder
2 tablespoons hulled hemp seed

Combine all ingredients in a high-power blender or food processor and blend until smooth. Drink immediately.

Serves 1

Nutrition Facts (per serving)

Calories 204
Fat 11 g
Carbs 26 g
Fiber 13 g
Protein 9 g

Sugimoto N, Miwa S, Hitomi Y, Nakamura H, Tsuchiya H, Yachie A. (2014) Theobromine, the Primary Methyl-xanthine Found in Theobroma cacao, Prevents Malignant Glioblastoma Proliferation by Negatively Regulating Phosphodiesterase-4, Extracellular Signal-regulated Kinase, Akt/mammalian Target of Rapamycin Kinase, and Nuclear Factor-Kappa B. *Nutrition and Cancer.*

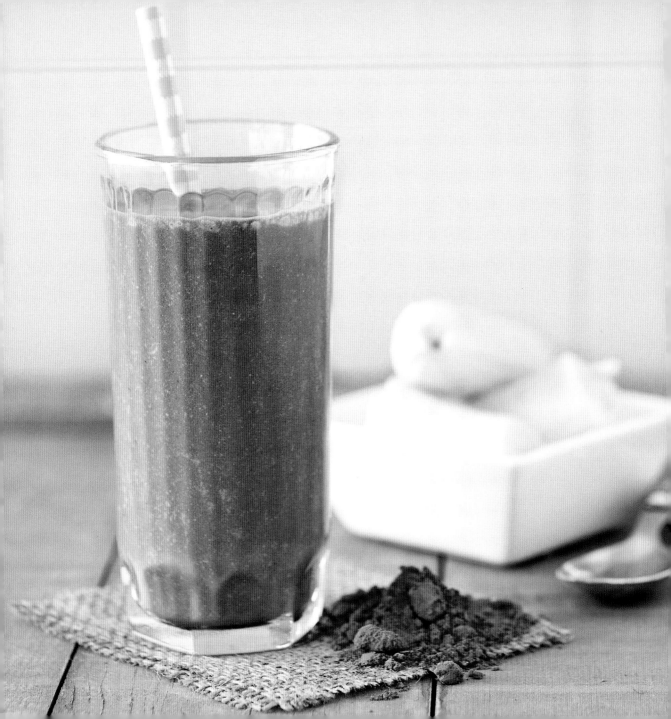

Banana Coconut Cocoa Cream

Cocoa is an excellent source of the mineral magnesium, which helps reduce inflammation and free radicals thus providing some protection against oxidative DNA damage that can lead to cancer development.

This creamy, comforting whip has distinctive cocoa, banana, and coconut flavors.

Ingredients

1 banana
1 cup cultured coconut milk
½ cup frozen white tea cubes
2 tablespoons unsweetened cocoa powder
2 tablespoons protein powder

Combine all ingredients in a high-power blender or food processor and blend until smooth. Drink immediately.

Serves 2

Nutrition Facts (per serving)

Calories 116
Fat 4 g
Carbs 15 g
Fiber 3 g
Protein 8 g

Blaszczyk U, Duda-Chodak A. (2013) Magnesium: its role in nutrition and carcinogenesis. *Rocz Panstw Zakl Hig.*

Chocolate Raspberry

Carrot intake increases the level of carotenoids in the blood and body tissues, which provides protection from cancer development.

This rich chocolate and berry smoothie has a fresh tea and cocoa fragrance.

Ingredients

½ cup carrot juice
½ cup frozen green tea cubes
½ cup frozen raspberries
2 tablespoons unsweetened cocoa powder
2 tablespoons protein powder

Combine all ingredients in a high-power blender or food processor and blend until smooth. Drink immediately.

Serves 1

Nutrition Facts (per serving)

Calories 251
Fat 2g
Carbs 42 g
Fiber 8 g
Protein 15 g

Xu X, Cheng Y, Li S, Zhu Y, Xu X, Zheng X, Mao Q, Xie L. (2014) Dietary carrot consumption and the risk of prostate cancer. *European Journal of Nutrition*.

Chocolate Vanilla Bean

Vanilla beans and real vanilla extract contain piperonal, which has the ability to cause apoptosis in several types of cancer including liver cancer.

With appetite stimulating vanilla fragrance, this frosty chocolate smoothie is as refreshing as it is light.

Ingredients

1 vanilla bean
1 cup green tea
½ cup cultured coconut milk
½ cup tangerine wedges
½ cup frozen grapes
2 tablespoons unsweetened cocoa powder
2 tablespoons protein powder

Combine all ingredients in a high-power blender or food processor and blend until smooth. Drink immediately.

Serves 2

Nutrition Facts (per serving)

Calories 126
Fat 2 g
Carbs 20 g
Fiber 3 g
Protein 8 g

Shi ZY, Li YQ, Kang YH, Hu GQ, Huang-fu CS, Deng JB, Liu B. (2012) Piperonal ciprofloxacin hydrazone induces growth arrest and apoptosis of human hepatocarcinoma SMMC-7721 cells. *Journal of the Chinese Pharmacological Society.*

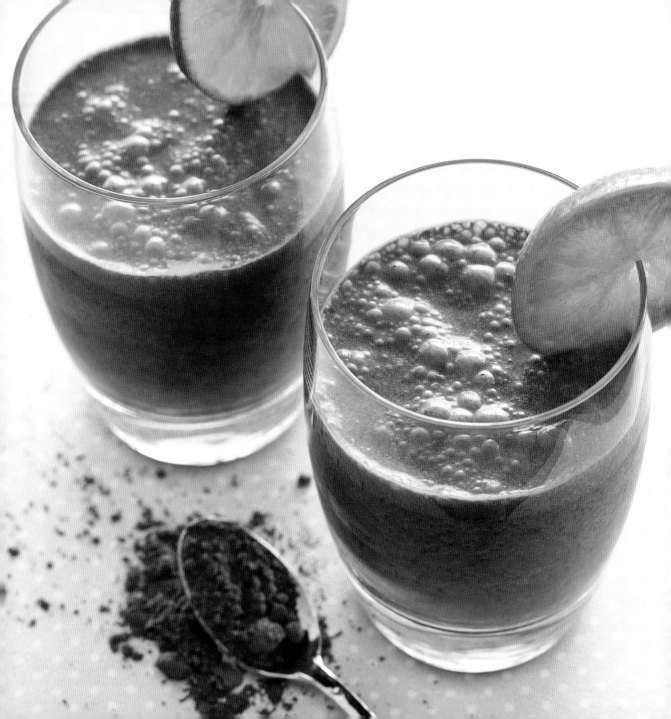

Cocoa Orange

Cryptoxanthin, a provitamin carotenoid in mandarin oranges, has proven to be effective at suppressing the growth and spread of stomach cancer cells in laboratory studies.

Fragrant with rich chocolate and orange scent, this smoothie is not too sweet and layered with rich flavors.

Ingredients

1 mandarin orange
1 frozen banana
½ cup orange juice
½ cup cultured coconut milk
½ cup frozen green tea cubes
2 tablespoons protein powder
2 tablespoons unsweetened cocoa powder

Combine all ingredients in a high-power blender or food processor and blend until smooth. Drink immediately.

Serves 2

Nutrition Facts (per serving)

Calories 183
Fat 3 g
Carbs 33 g
Fiber 4 g
Protein 9 g

Wu C, Han L, Riaz H, Wang S, Cai K, Yang L. (2013) The chemopreventive effect of β-cryptoxanthin from mandarin on human stomach cells (BGC-823). *Food Chemistry*.

Banana Chocolate Cream

Cocoa is rich in theobromine and epicatechins, which have anticancer properties as they interact with specific molecular targets linked to the development of cancer.

This smoothie is rich and tastes like soft-serve, semisweet, chocolate ice cream.

Ingredients

1 frozen banana
1 cup cultured coconut
   milk
2 tablespoons hulled
   hemp seed
1 tablespoon unsweetened
   cocoa powder

Combine all ingredients in a high-power blender or food processor and blend until smooth. Drink immediately.

Serves 1

Nutrition Facts (per serving)

Calories 212
Fat 6 g
Carbs 27 g
Fiber 5 g
Protein 14 g

Kim J, Shim J, Lee CY, Lee KW, Lee HJ. (2014) Cocoa phytochemicals: recent advances in molecular mechanisms on health. *Critical Reviews in Food Science and Nutrition*.

Mexican Cocoa

Cayenne pepper contains capsaicin that has the ability to induce apoptosis of cancer cells.

Cocoa, cinnamon, and cayenne flavors add depth to this rich and creamy combination of banana, hemp, and almond milk.

Ingredients

1 frozen banana
½ cup almond milk
2 tablespoons hulled
  hemp seed
1 tablespoon unsweetened
  cocoa powder
1 teaspoon cinnamon
Pinch of cayenne pepper

Combine all ingredients in a high-power blender or food processor and blend until smooth. Drink immediately.

Serves 1

Nutrition Facts (per serving)

Calories 259
Fat 11 g
Carbs 39 g
Fiber 14 g
Protein 9 g

Anandakumar P, Kamaraj S, Jagan S, Ramakrishnan G, Devaki T. (2013) Capsaicin provokes apoptosis and restricts benzo(a)pyrene induced lung tumorigenesis in Swiss albino mice. *International Immunopharmacology.*

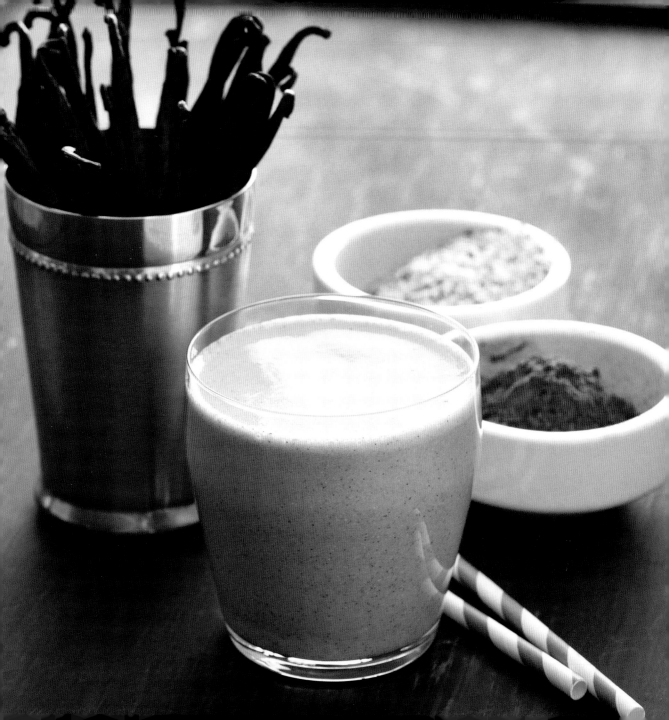

Chocolate Vanilla Bean Cream

Anthocyanins are major flavonoids found in cocoa that have the ability to reduce the growth and spread of cancer cells. Probiotics in cultured coconut milk enhance the absorption and activity of these nutrients from cocoa when they are ingested together.

This chocolate and coconut combination has exotic vanilla bean flavor.

Ingredients

½ cup cultured coconut milk
½ cup frozen green tea cubes
1 tablespoon unsweetened cocoa powder
1 tablespoon hulled hemp seed
1 vanilla bean

Combine all ingredients in a high-power blender or food processor and blend until smooth. Drink immediately.

Serves 1

Nutrition Facts (per serving)

Calories 105
Fat 8 g
Carbs 10 g
Fiber 8 g
Protein 4 g

Fernandes I, Marques F, de Freitas V, Mateus N. (2013) Antioxidant and antiproliferative properties of methylated metabolites of anthocyanins. *Food Chemistry.*

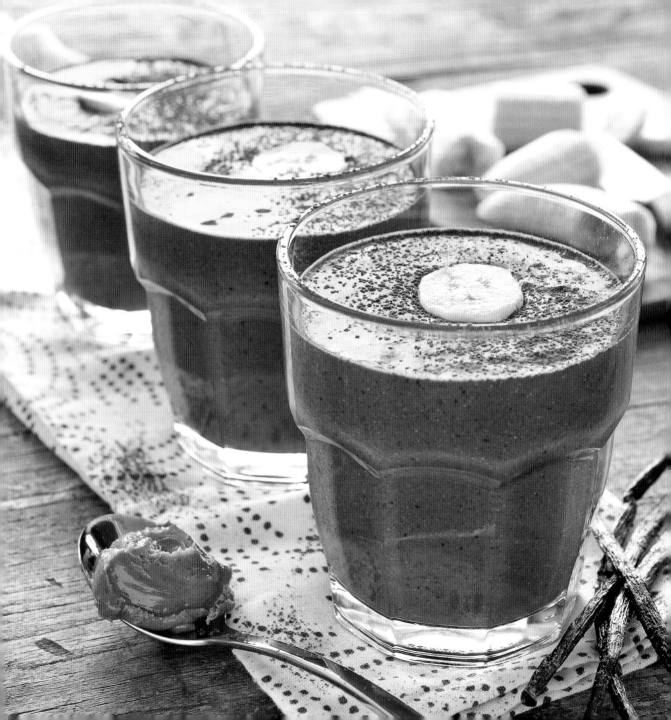

Banana Split

Resveratrol, found in peanuts and peanut butter, has been found to suppress intestinal cancers.

The cocoa and vanilla fragrances stimulate the appetite while the peanut butter and vanilla bean flavor hit the palate. The taste is reminiscent of slightly melted chocolate ice cream.

Ingredients

1 frozen banana
1 vanilla bean
1 cup almond milk
½ cup frozen cherries
2 tablespoons peanut
    butter
2 tablespoons vanilla
    protein powder
2 tablespoons hulled
    hemp seed
2 tablespoons
    unsweetened cocoa
    powder

Combine all ingredients in a high-power blender or food processor and blend until smooth. Drink immediately.

Serves 2

Nutrition Facts (per serving)

Calories 295
Fat 15 g
Carbs 30 g
Fiber 9 g
Protein 15 g

Altamemi I, Murphy EA, Catroppo JF, Zumbrun EE, Zhang J, McClellan JL, Singh UP, Nagarkatti PS, Nagarkatti M. (2014) Role of microRNAs in resveratrol-mediated mitigation of colitis-associated tumorigenesis in ApcMin/+ mice. *Journal of Pharmacology and Experimental Therapeutics*.

Herbal Smoothies

Ginger root contains natural compounds including shogaol, allicin, diallyl trisulfide, and vanilloids which produce chemopreventive, anti-inflammatory, and anticancer properties. The juice adds a flavor and a warming quality to smoothies.

Garlic enhances our immunity against cancer by boosting the functioning of the immune system, activating immune specialized cells that eventually lead to improvement in the defense system, and inducing apoptosis.

Cardamom contains limonene and cineole, which are phytochemicals that act against carcinogenesis.

Holy basil leaves inhibit the proliferation, migration, and invasion of pancreatic cancer cells and induce apoptosis.

Rosemary provides rosmarinic and carnosic acid, which are shown to prevent radiation-induced DNA damage.

Turmeric contains curcumin, a natural compound with the ability to arrest the cell cycle and induce apoptosis in cancer cells.

Piperine, a major alkaloid constituent of black pepper, has diverse physiological actions including apoptosis and acts as an angiogenesis inhibitor.

Black pepper and cardamom, when ingested together, help regulate inflammation and prevent carcinogenesis.

Also, some greens contain important medicinal oils. For example, spinach has a natural antioxidant mixture that directly reduces cancer growth and development.

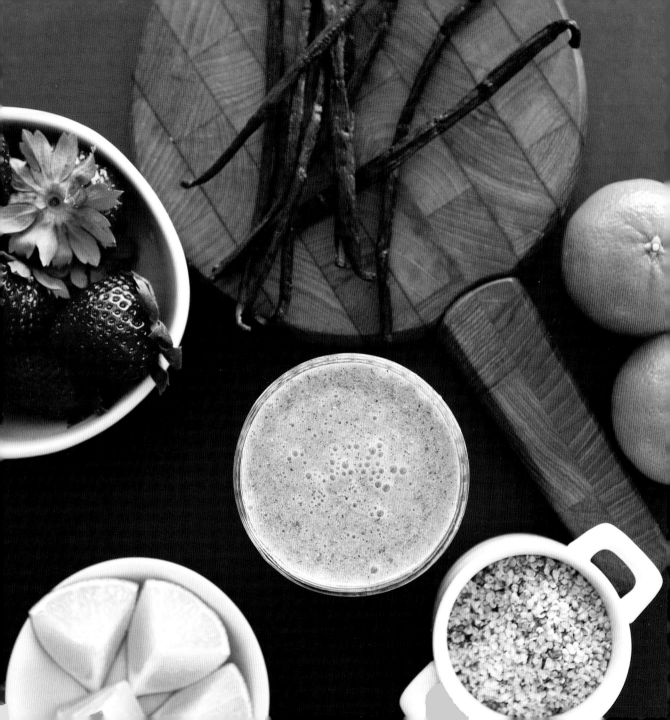

Vanilla Berry Lime

Vanilla contains vanillin, which directly reduces cancer growth and development.

This citrus and berry smoothie is sweet and tart and tastes a bit like candy but less sweet as it is tempered by the tea and hemp protein.

Ingredients

1 lime wedge
1 vanilla bean
½ cup tangerine
½ cup pomegranate juice
½ cup frozen strawberries
½ cup cultured coconut milk
½ cup frozen green tea cubes
2 tablespoons hulled hemp seed

Combine all ingredients in a high-power blender or food processor and blend until smooth. Drink immediately.

Serves 2

Nutrition Facts (per serving)

Calories 143
Fat 6 g
Carbs 24 g
Fiber 8 g
Protein 4 g

Khuda-Bukhsh AR, Das S, Saha SK. (2014) Molecular approaches toward targeted cancer prevention with some food plants and their products: inflammatory and other signal pathways. *Nutrition and Cancer.*

Vanilla Lime Mango

Vanilla beans and vanilla extracts contain vanillin, which is anti-metastatic and anti-angiogenic.

A sweet mango base with exotic vanilla bean and lime flavor, this smoothie has French vanilla flecks.

Ingredients
1 lime wedge
1 vanilla bean
½ cup currant juice
½ cup frozen mango
½ cup frozen green tea
  cubes
2 tablespoons vanilla
  protein powder

Combine all ingredients in a high-power blender or food processor and blend until smooth. Drink immediately.

Serves 1

Nutrition Facts (per serving)

Calories 126
Fat 0 g
Carbs 17 g
Fiber 2 g
Protein 13 g

Lirdprapamongkol K, Sakurai H, Suzuki S, Koizumi K, Prangsaengtong O, Viriyaroj A, Ruchirawat S, Svasti J, Saiki I. (2010) Vanillin enhances TRAIL-induced apoptosis in cancer cells through inhibition of NF-kappaB activation. *In Vivo.*

Pineapple and Holy Basil

Holy basil contains several anticancer phytochemicals including eugenol, rosmarinic acid, apigenin, myretenal, luteolin, β-sitosterol, and carnosic acid which increase antioxidant activity, alter gene expression, induce apoptosis, and inhibit angiogenesis and metastasis.

Rich and frosty, this combination has intense pineapple and currant flavor.

Ingredients

½ cup currant juice
½ cup frozen strawberries
½ cup frozen green tea cubes
½ cup frozen pineapple
½ cup orange juice
¼ cup fresh holy basil leaves
2 tablespoons hulled hemp seed

Combine all ingredients in a high-power blender or food processor and blend until smooth. Drink immediately.

Serves 2

Nutrition Facts (per serving)

Calories 128
Fat 5 g
Carbs 22 g
Fiber 7 g
Protein 4 g

Baliga MS, Jimmy R, Thilakchand KR, Sunitha V, Bhat NR, Saldanha E, Rao S, Rao P, Arora R, Palatty PL. (2013) Ocimum sanctum L (Holy Basil or Tulsi) and its phytochemicals in the prevention and treatment of cancer. *Nutrition and Cancer.*

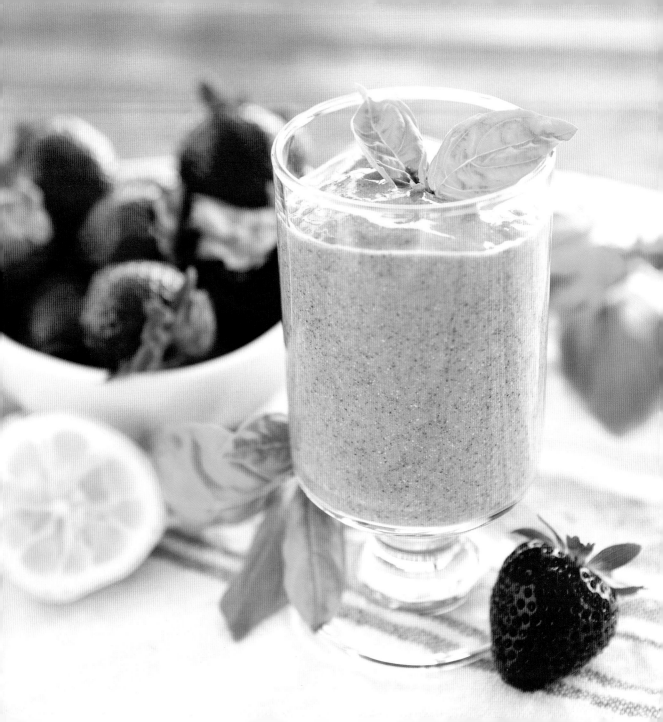

Strawberry and Basil Lemonade

Basil contains powerful antioxidants that protect against cellular damage and provide proven protection against breast cancer development.

This light smoothie has a fresh basil fragrance and sweet strawberry flavor with a citrus finish.

Ingredients

½ cup strawberries
½ cup fresh basil leaves
½ cup water
½ cup frozen green tea cubes
2 tablespoons chia seed
1 tablespoon lemon juice

Combine all ingredients in a high-power blender or food processor and blend until smooth. Drink immediately.

Serves 1

Nutrition Facts (per serving)

Calories 166
Fat 10 g
Carbs 8 g
Fiber 14 g
Protein 7 g

Al-Ali KH, El-Beshbishy HA, El-Badry AA, Alkhalaf M. (2013) Cytotoxic activity of methanolic extract of Mentha longifolia and Ocimum basilicum against human breast cancer. *Pakistan Journal of Biological Sciences*.

Rosemary Elixir

Bromelain from pineapple is a rich source of metabolic enzymes that slow the growth and spread of cancer cells by inducing apoptosis.

A brilliant pink color, this unique blend is brisk with a pine-like aroma and a complex, sweet flavor.

Ingredients

½ cup pineapple
½ cup pomegranate juice
½ cup frozen green tea
  cubes
2 tablespoons fresh
  rosemary
2 tablespoons hulled
  hemp seed

Combine all ingredients in a high-power blender or food processor and blend until smooth. Drink immediately.

Serves 1

Nutrition Facts (per serving)

Calories 244
Fat 9 g
Carbs 41 g
Fiber 12 g
Protein 6 g

Amini A, Ehteda A, Masoumi Moghaddam S, Akhter J, Pillai K, Morris DL.(2013) Cytotoxic effects of bromelain in human gastrointestinal carcinoma cell lines (MKN45, KATO-III, HT29-5F12, and HT29-5M21). *Oncology Targets and Therapy.*

Tangerine Currant

Citrus peel oil contains tangeretin, a nutrient compound that has the ability to induce apoptosis in breast, colorectal, and lung cancers.

The tangerine tang and lush currant flavor are a mouthwatering and fresh combination.

Ingredients

1 lemon wedge
½ cup tangerine
½ cup currant juice
½ cup frozen green tea cubes
2 tablespoons hulled hemp seed
1 tablespoon fresh rosemary

Combine all ingredients in a high-power blender or food processor and blend until smooth. Drink immediately.

Serves 1

Nutrition Facts (per serving)

Calories 171
Fat 9 g
Carbs 23 g
Fiber 12 g
Protein 7 g

Dong Y, Cao A, Shi J, Yin P, Wang L, Ji G, Xie J, Wu D. (2014) Tangeretin, a citrus polymethoxyflavonoid, induces apoptosis of human gastric cancer AGS cells through extrinsic and intrinsic signaling pathways. *Oncology Reports.*

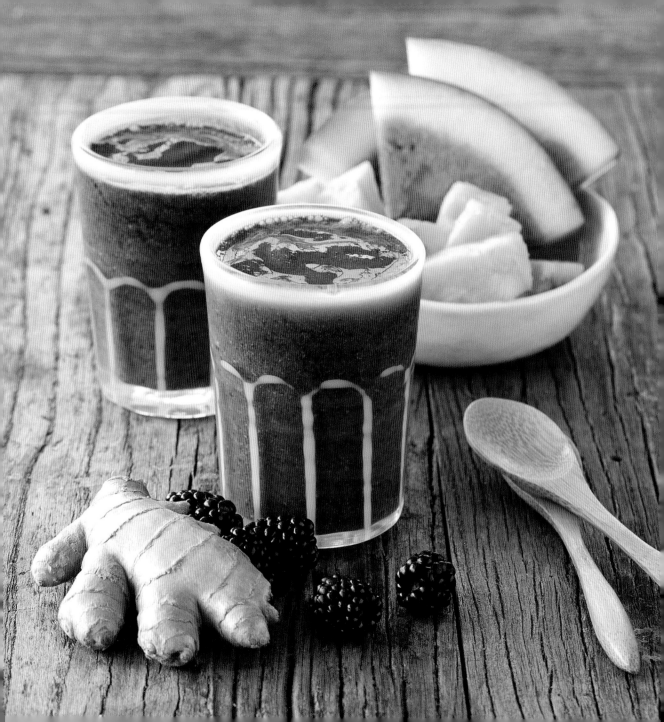

Watermelon Blackberry and Ginger

Ginger contains gingerol, which is the major pungent component of ginger. Gingerol reduces cancer growth by inhibiting the metastatic process.

This smoothie has fresh watermelon and blackberry flavor with a little bit of heat from the ginger.

Ingredients

½ cup orange juice
½ cup watermelon
½ cup frozen blackberries
½ cup frozen pineapple
½ cup frozen green tea cubes
2 tablespoons hulled hemp seed
1 tablespoon fresh ginger root

Combine all ingredients in a high-power blender or food processor and blend until smooth. Drink immediately.

Serves 2

Nutrition Facts (per serving)

Calories 158
Fat 5 g
Carbs 29 g
Fiber 9 g
Protein 5 g

Poltronieri J, Becceneri AB, Fuzer AM, C Filho JC, B M Martin AC, Vieira PC, Pouliot N, Cominetti MR. Mini Rev Med Chem. (2014) [6]-gingerol as a Cancer Chemopreventive Agent: A Review of Its Activity on Different Steps of the Metastatic Process. *Mini-Reviews in Medicinal Chemistry.*

Blackberry Citrus and Holy Basil

Holy basil, which is also known as tulsi, has been found to provide protection against the development of cancer as well as reducing existing cancer cells.

This smoothie has a rich blackberry flavor and light holy basil fragrance.

Ingredients

½ cup frozen green tea cubes
½ cup frozen blackberries
¼ cup carrot juice
¼ cup orange juice
¼ cup fresh holy basil leaves
2 tablespoons hulled hemp seeds

Combine all ingredients in a high-power blender or food processor and blend until smooth. Drink immediately.

Serves 1

Nutrition Facts (per serving)

Calories 213
Fat 9 g
Carbs 31 g
Fiber 16 g
Protein 8 g

Bhattacharyya P, Bishayee A. (2013) Ocimum sanctum Linn. (Tulsi): an ethnomedicinal plant for the prevention and treatment of cancer. *Anticancer Drugs*.

Watermelon Pom and Holy Basil

Holy basil provides protection and healing via its natural compounds that reduce inflammation, reduce stress, and support the immune system.

The fragrance of holy basil, in this fresh watermelon and pomegranate smoothie, stimulates the appetite while the sweetness is grounded in an earthy hemp and green tea base.

Ingredients

½ cup pomegranate seeds
½ cup watermelon
½ cup fresh holy basil leaves
¼ cup frozen green tea cubes
¼ cup tart cherry juice
¼ cup carrot juice
2 tablespoons hulled hemp seed
1 tablespoon lemon juice

Combine all ingredients in a high-power blender or food processor and blend until smooth. Drink immediately.

Serves 2

Nutrition Facts (per serving)

Calories 138
Fat 5
Carbs 23 g
Fiber 7 g
Protein 4 g

Baliga MS, Jimmy R, Thilakchand KR, Sunitha V, Bhat NR, Saldanha E, Rao S, Rao P, Arora R, Palatty PL. (2013) Ocimum sanctum L (Holy Basil or Tulsi) and its phytochemicals in the prevention and treatment of cancer. *Nutrition and Cancer.*

Peel Power

Recent research is focusing on the anticancer compounds in the edible peels and skins of fruits such as apples, citrus fruits, and bananas.

Apple skins contain nutrient phytochemicals, including flavonoids (catechins, flavonols, and quercetin) and phenolic acids (quercetin glycosides, catechin, epicatechin, and procyanidins), vitamins, and fibers, which reduce the growth of cancer cells. These anti-proliferative compounds are also found in the apple's interior but are so concentrated in the skin that researchers are creating extracts from them to use as cancer treatment.

Flavonoids in citrus fruits (pulp and juice), such as tangeretin, that trigger apoptosis in cancer cells are also found in the oils of the peel. Adding small amounts of citrus peel, about two tablespoons per smoothie, boosts these anticancer nutrients while providing intense citrus flavor and mouthwatering citrus fragrance to smoothies.

Banana peels also contain concentrated amounts of the same powerful, antioxidant phenolics as the fruit. For example, the dopamine found in bananas is highly concentrated in the peel. Keep in mind that only organic banana peel is edible. Non-organic bananas have been found to have an unhealthy residue of toxic compounds.

Citrus fruit peels may add cancer fighting compounds to smoothies, but too much peel may add more fiber and bitter flavor than is palatable. As a general guideline, adding about two tablespoons of peel to each recipe will provide an effective dose of tangeretin. This amount replicates the amount given to the animals in the studies, which comprises about 1 percent of the diet.

If you have a high-power blender, you will be able to add as much peel and skin as you'd like and it will blend easily. If your blender struggles with fiber, start by adding small amounts of peel; for example, add a lemon wedge to see if it will blend. If not, simply leave the skins, rinds, and peels out and use the fruit segments, juice, and citrus oils.

Pom Lime Wedge

Resveratrol is a natural polyphenol found in grapes that acts as an anti-inflammatory and anticancer agent.

This smoothie has a sweet, rich, grape flavor, yet the tea keeps it from being too sweet and the lime wedge adds both tartness and a heady fragrance of essential oil.

Ingredients

2 lime wedges
½ cup pomegranate juice
½ cup frozen red grapes
½ cup frozen green tea cubes
2 tablespoons hulled hemp seed

Combine all ingredients in a high-power blender or food processor and blend until smooth. Drink immediately.

Serves 2

Nutrition Facts (per serving)

Calories 133
Fat 5 g
Carbs 24 g
Fiber 6 g
Protein 4 g

Gambini J, López-Grueso R, Olaso-González G, Inglés M, Abdelazid K, El Alami M, Bonet-Costa V, Borrás C, Viña J. (2013) Resveratrol: distribution, properties and perspectives. *Review Spanish Geriatrics & Gerontology.*

Tangerine Lemon Wedge

Tangeretin in citrus peel oil has proven to cause apoptosis (cancer cell destruction) in breast cancer, colorectal carcinoma, and lung carcinoma studies.

This tangy smoothie is mouthwatering with a balance of sweet, sour, and bitter that leaves you wanting more.

Ingredients

1 lemon wedge
½ cup pomegranate juice
½ cup tangerine
½ cup frozen strawberries
½ cup frozen green tea
 cubes
2 tablespoons hulled
 hemp seed

Combine all ingredients in a high-power blender or food processor and blend until smooth. Drink immediately.

Serves 2

Nutrition Facts (per serving)

Calories 116
Fat 3
Carbs 19
Fiber 3
Protein 3

Tundis R, Loizzo MR, Menichini F. (2014) An overview on chemical aspects and potential health benefits of limonoids and their derivatives. *Critical Reviews in Food Science and Nutrition.*

Blood Orange and Blackberry

Blood oranges contain concentrated amounts of tangeretin, a natural plant compound that triggers apoptosis in cancer cells.

This blackberry and blood orange blend has bold citrus flavor and fragrance complemented by lime essence.

Ingredients

1 lime wedge
½ cup frozen blackberries
½ cup blood orange
½ cup frozen green tea cubes
½ cup green tea
2 tablespoons hulled hemp seed

Combine all ingredients in a high-power blender or food processor and blend until smooth. Drink immediately.

Serves 1

Nutrition Facts (per serving)

Calories 190
Fat 7 g
Carbs 27 g
Fiber 10 g
Protein 7 g

Dong Y, Cao A, Shi J, Yin P, Wang L, Ji G, Xie J, Wu D. (2014) Tangeretin, a citrus polymethoxyflavonoid, induces apoptosis of human gastric cancer AGS cells through extrinsic and intrinsic signaling pathways. *Oncology Reports.*

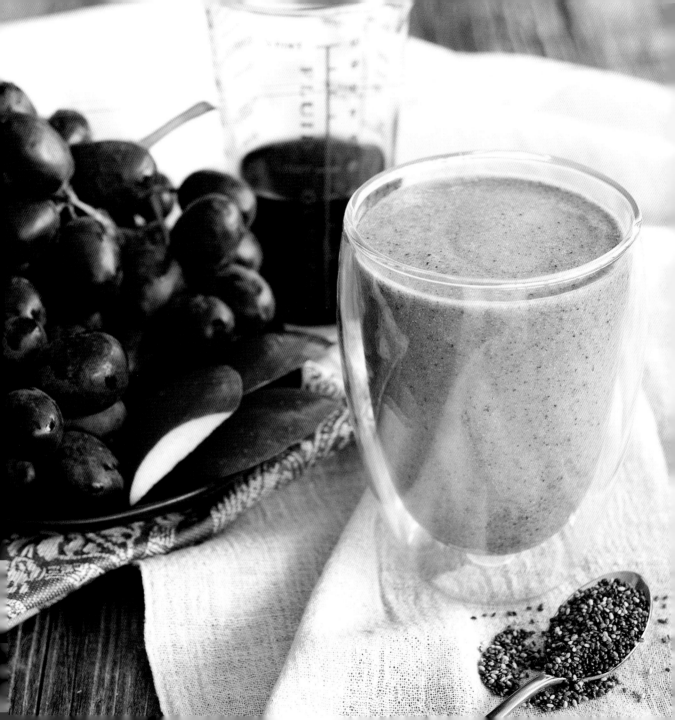

Currant Lime Wedge

The peel of the lime contains tangeretin, a flavonoid that triggers apoptosis in many types of cancer.

Bold currant flavor, sweetened with fresh watermelon, this combination is punctuated with tart lime flavor and fresh lime essence.

Ingredients

1 lime wedge
½ cup currant juice
½ cup watermelon
½ cup frozen green tea cubes
2 tablespoons hulled hemp seed

Combine all ingredients in a high-power blender or food processor and blend until smooth. Drink immediately.

Serves 1

Nutrition Facts (per serving)

Calories 125
Fat 6 g
Carbs 12 g
Fiber 2 g
Protein 6 g

Dong Y, Cao A, Shi J, Yin P, Wang L, Ji G, Xie J, Wu D. (2014) Tangeretin, a citrus polymethoxyflavonoid, induces apoptosis of human gastric cancer AGS cells through extrinsic and intrinsic signaling pathways. *Oncology Reports*.

Blood Orange and Lime Wedge

Blood oranges provide antioxidant carotenoids, which reduce the risk for development of cancer as we age via their antioxidant effects.

Coconut and sweet citrus mingle in this delicious smoothie blend.

Ingredients

1 lime wedge
½ cup blood orange
½ cup watermelon
½ cup cultured coconut milk
½ cup frozen white tea cubes
2 tablespoons hulled hemp seed

Combine all ingredients in a high-power blender or food processor and blend until smooth. Drink immediately.

Serves 1

Nutrition Facts (per serving)

Calories 198
Fat 9 g
Carbs 26 g
Fiber 5 g
Protein 7 g

Woodside JV, McGrath AJ, Lyner N, McKinley MC. (2015) Carotenoids and health in older people. *Maturitas.*

Piña Colada

Oranges and pineapple contain melatonin, which is an important antioxidant that interferes with the development of many types of cancer.

This smoothie might make you feel like you're on a mini-vacation with its sweet and tangy pineapple flavor, coconut nibbles, and tropical fragrance.

Ingredients

1 lime wedge
1 cup orange juice
½ cup frozen green tea cubes
½ cup pineapple
2 tablespoons shredded unsweetened coconut
2 tablespoons hulled hemp seed

Combine all ingredients in a high-power blender or food processor and blend until smooth. Drink immediately.

Serves 2

Nutrition Facts (per serving)

Calories 222
Fat 12 g
Carbs 25 g
Fiber 4 g
Protein 5 g

Sae-Teaw M, Johns J, Johns NP, Subongkot S. (2013) Serum melatonin levels and antioxidant capacities after consumption of pineapple, orange, or banana by healthy male volunteers. *Journal of Pineal Research*.

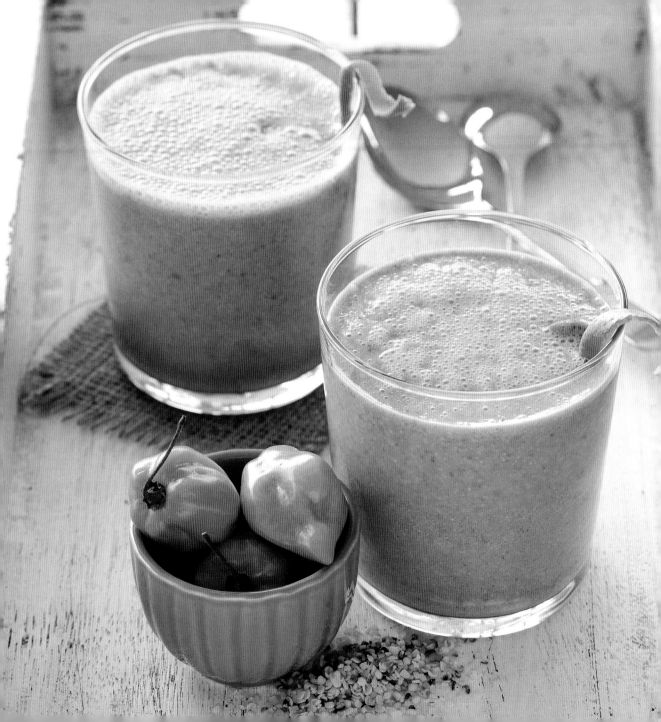

Habanero and Citrus

Tangeretin is a naturally occurring plant compound found in significant amounts in the peel of citrus fruits. Tangeretin dramatically reduced breast cancer cells in lab studies and repeated studies have found that tangeretin is effective at causing apoptosis in many types of cancer.

Ice-cold and spicy hot, this combination has a hot pepper bite and a light citrus note with sweet berry and bitter orange.

Ingredients

¼ orange
¼ small habanero pepper
½ cup watermelon
½ cup frozen green tea cubes
½ cup frozen strawberries
2 tablespoons hulled hemp seed

Combine all ingredients in a high-power blender or food processor and blend until smooth. Drink immediately.

Serves 2

Nutrition Facts (per serving)

Calories 87
Fat 3 g
Carbs 12 g
Fiber 4 g
Protein 3 g

Lakshmi A, Subramanian S. (2014) Chemotherapeutic effect of tangeretin, a polymethoxylated flavone studied in 7, 12-dimethylbenz(a)anthracene induced mammary carcinoma in experimental rats. *Biochimie*.

Banana Healer

Banana peels contain compounds with anticancer benefits for those with prostate cancer.

Creamy and sweet, this tropical citrus smoothie has complex flavor thanks to the pineapple, strawberry, and banana.

Ingredients

½ banana
½ cup orange juice
½ cup frozen pineapple
½ frozen strawberries
2 tablespoons hulled
   hemp seed

Combine all ingredients in a high-power blender or food processor and blend until smooth. Drink immediately.

Serves 2

Nutrition Facts (per serving)

Calories 135
Fat 3 g
Carbs 24 g
Fiber 4 g
Protein 4 g

Akamine K, Koyama T, Yazawa K. (2009) Banana peel extract suppressed prostate gland enlargement in testosterone-treated mice. *Bioscience, Biotechnology and Biochemistry*.

Golden Berry Apple

Apples are rich in phenolic acids that inhibit cancer by reducing the growth of cancer and even reversing it, thereby reducing the risk for development of invasive cancers.

This simple combination has sweet blueberry and apple flavor and nutrient–rich plant fiber.

Ingredients

½ apple
1 cup frozen wild blueberries
½ cup unfiltered apple juice
2 tablespoons hulled hemp seed
½ teaspoon turmeric powder

Combine all ingredients in a high-power blender or food processor and blend until smooth. Drink immediately.

Serves 2

Nutrition Facts (per serving)

Calories 148
Fat 3 g
Carbs 29 g
Fiber 7 g
Protein 3 g

Ribeiro FA, Gomes de Moura CF, Aguiar O Jr, de Oliveira F, Spadari RC, Oliveira NR, Oshima CT, Ribeiro DA. (2013) The chemopreventive activity of apple against carcinogenesis: antioxidant activity and cell cycle control. *European Journal of Cancer Prevention.*

Protein Power

Boost the protein and calories in your smoothies by increasing the amount of protein powder, chia seed, hulled hemp seed, and nut butter you use. Aim for a minimum of 60 grams of dietary protein intake per day.

Whole-food sources of protein that blend well in smoothies are chia seed and hulled hemp seed, as they not only provide protein but fiber and essential fatty acids as well. Hemp and chia provide omega-3 fatty acids, which appear to exert their anticancer actions by influencing multiple targets implicated in various stages of cancer development, including cell proliferation, cell survival, angiogenesis, inflammation, metastasis, and epigenetic abnormalities.

Protein powders provide amino acids that reduce the loss of muscle mass and the development of cachexia. Protein powders blend easily into smoothies and most are highly digestible. Plant-based powders are made from plant foods such as peas, rice, seeds, and hemp. Dairy-based powders such as whey should be avoided as they are contraindicated for many types of cancer. The plain protein powders are the lowest in sugar and the vanilla-flavored are generally fairly low in sugar while providing vanilla flavor and fragrance, which is why I often choose the vanilla-flavored powders.

Pom Pine

Urolithins are bioactive metabolites in pomegranate that are produced by our gut flora from ellagitannins and ellagic acid. Our natural gut flora helps metabolize these cancer-preventive nutrients from pomegranates (seeds and juice).

Sweet pineapple and slightly tart pomegranate pair perfectly in this light smoothie. This is one of my favorite daily smoothies for its flavor and nutrient benefits.

Ingredients

½ cup pomegranate juice
½ cup frozen green tea cubes
½ cup fresh pineapple
2 tablespoons protein powder

Combine all ingredients in a high-power blender or food processor and blend until smooth. Drink immediately.

Serves 1

Nutrition Facts (per serving)

Calories 182
Fat 0 g
Carbs 31 g
Fiber 2 g
Protein 13 g

Nuñez-Sánchez MA, García-Villalba R, Monedero-Saiz T, García-Talavera NV, Gómez-Sánchez MB, Sánchez-Álvarez C, García-Albert AM, Rodríguez-Gil FJ, Ruiz-Marín M, Pastor-Quirante FA, Martínez-Díaz F, Yáñez-Gascón MJ, González-Sarrías A, Tomás-Barberán FA, Espín JC. (2014) Targeted metabolic profiling of pomegranate polyphenols and urolithins in plasma, urine and colon tissues from colorectal cancer patients. *Molecular Nutrition & Food Research*.

Orange Berry Sherbet

Green tea provides protection from cancer and reduces blood pressure and cholesterol levels.

This bright, intense, citrus and berry smoothie is slightly tart, which gives it a sherbet-like flavor.

Ingredients

½ cup orange juice
½ cup frozen red
  raspberries
½ cup frozen green tea
  cubes
2 tablespoons protein
  powder

Combine all ingredients in a high-power blender or food processor and blend until smooth. Drink immediately.

Serves 1

Nutrition Facts (per serving)

Calories 172
Fat 1 g
Carbs 27 g
Fiber 8 g
Protein 14 g

Onakpoya I, Spencer E, Heneghan C, Thompson M. (2014) The effect of green tea on blood pressure and lipid profile: A systematic review and meta-analysis of randomized clinical trials. *Nutrition Metabolism and Cardiovascular Disease.*

Grapefruit and Green Tea

Grapefruit provides kaempferol, which protects against cardiovascular disease and metastatic cancer growth.

Light, cool, and creamy, this peach and green tea smoothie has a refreshing hint of tart grapefruit.

Ingredients

¼ cup grapefruit
½ cup frozen peaches
½ cup frozen green tea cubes
½ cup filtered water
2 tablespoons protein powder

Combine all ingredients in a high-power blender or food processor and blend until smooth. Drink immediately.

Serves 1

Nutrition Facts (per serving)

Calories 112
Fat 0 g
Carbs 13 g
Fiber 1 g
Protein 13 g

Lin CW, Chen PN, Chen MK, Yang WE, Tang CH, Yang SF, Hsieh YS. (2013) Kaempferol reduces matrix metalloproteinase-2 expression by down-regulating ERK ½ and the activator protein-1 signaling pathways in oral cancer cells. *PLoS One.*

Vanilla Berry Cream

Weight loss—particularly muscle weight loss—weakens the body's ability to heal from cancer. Daily intake of amino acids in the form of dietary protein from easily digestible, whole-food sources such as protein powders, hulled hemp seed, and chia seed, can reduce this muscle weight loss.

This smoothie has rich berry citrus flavor with a heady fragrance of vanilla and flecks of vanilla bean.

Ingredients

1 vanilla bean
½ cup orange juice
½ cup frozen red raspberries
½ cup frozen green tea cubes
2 tablespoons protein powder

Combine all ingredients in a high-power blender or food processor and blend until smooth. Drink immediately.

Serves 1

Nutrition Facts (per serving)

Calories 231
Fat 0 g
Carbs 43 g
Fiber 5 g
Protein 14 g

Al-Zhoughbi W, Huang J, Paramasivan GS, Till H, Pichler M, Guertl-Lackner B, Hoefler G. (2014) Tumor macroenvironment and metabolism. *Seminars in Oncology*.

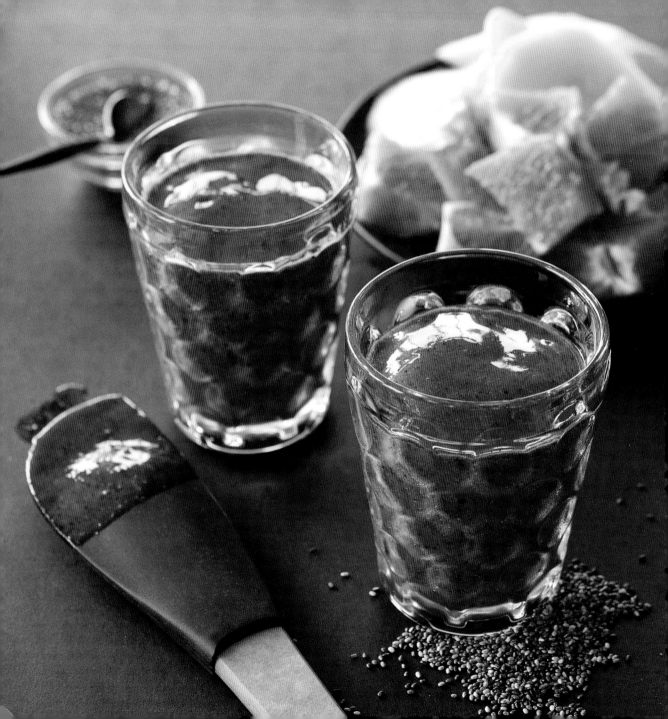

Mango Citrus

The antitumor activities of polyphenols, such as ellagitannins and anthocyanins in pomegranate, are anti-inflammatory and cytotoxic against colon cancer.

Mango gives this smoothie a rich and creamy base while the citrus brightens the intense flavor of the pomegranate juice.

Ingredients

½ cup pomegranate juice
½ cup orange
½ cup mango
½ cup frozen green tea cubes
2 tablespoons chia seed

Combine all ingredients in a high-power blender or food processor and blend until smooth. Drink immediately.

Serves 2

Nutrition Facts (per serving)

Calories 163
Fat 5 g
Carbs 24 g
Fiber 8 g
Protein 4 g

Banerjee N, Kim H, Talcott S, Mertens-Talcott S. (2013) Pomegranate polyphenolics suppressed azoxymethane-induced colorectal aberrant crypt foci and inflammation: possible role of miR-126/VCAM-1 and miR-126/PI3K/AKT/mTOR. *Carcinogenesis*.

Grape Pom Pineapple

Ellagitannins are bioactive polyphenols in pomegranate juice that have anticancer properties found to be effective against prostate cancer. Ellagitannins are created when the ellagic acid in pomegranate juice is converted in the gut by the healthy bacteria that cover the intestinal walls. These compounds dramatically decrease cancer cell growth.

This simple, pink smoothie is rich in grape and pineapple flavor.

Ingredients

½ cup pomegranate juice
½ cup fresh pineapple
½ cup frozen grapes
½ cup frozen green tea
   cubes
2 tablespoons protein
   powder

Combine all ingredients in a high-power blender or food processor and blend until smooth. Drink immediately.

Serves 2

Nutrition Facts (per serving)

Calories 130
Fat 0 g
Carbs 26 g
Fiber 1 g
Protein 7 g

Vicinanza R, Zhang Y, Henning SM, Heber D. (2013) Pomegranate Juice Metabolites, Ellagic Acid and Urolithin A, Synergistically Inhibit Androgen-Independent Prostate Cancer Cell Growth via Distinct Effects on Cell Cycle Control and Apoptosis. *Evidence Based Complementary Alternative Medicine.*

Healing Smoothies

Grape Berry Citrus

Hulled hemp seed is nutrient-rich, providing 3 grams of healthful essential fatty acids, 3 grams of protein, and 1 gram of fiber in each tablespoon.

This pink berry blend is sweet with a little tart citrus flavor.

Ingredients

½ cup green tea
½ cup orange
½ cup frozen grapes
½ cup frozen strawberries
2 tablespoons hulled
   hemp seed
1 tablespoon lemon juice

Combine all ingredients in a high-power blender or food processor and blend until smooth. Drink immediately.

Serves 2

Nutrition Facts (per serving)

Calories 122
Fat 3 g
Carbs 21 g
Fiber 3 g
Protein 4 g

Crisp Cranberry

Cranberry juice contains myrecitin, which reduces cancer development through epigenetics and by directly minimizing inflammation.

The sweet grapes balance the tart cranberry in this fresh, tea–based, watermelon smoothie.

Ingredients

1 cup frozen white tea
  cubes
½ cup watermelon
½ cup frozen grapes
¼ cup cranberry juice
2 tablespoons chia seed

Combine all ingredients in a high-power blender or food processor and blend until smooth. Drink immediately.

Serves 2

Nutrition Facts (per serving)

Calories 141
Fat 5 g
Carbs 20 g
Fiber 7 g
Protein 4 g

Khuda-Bukhsh AR, Das S, Saha SK. (2014) Molecular approaches toward targeted cancer prevention with some food plants and their products: inflammatory and other signal pathways. *Nutrition and Cancer.*

Hemp Berry Citrus

Omega-3 fatty acids found in hemp seed, particularly eicosapentaenoic acid (EPA) and docosahexaenoic acid (DHA), exert anticancer actions by influencing various stages of cancer development including cell proliferation, cell survival, angiogenesis, inflammation, metastasis, and epigenetic abnormalities that can lead to cancer.

The lime wedge in this smoothie gives the blend a tangy citrus hit that balances the currant and raspberry flavors well.

Ingredients

1 lime wedge
1 cup currant juice
½ cup frozen raspberries
½ cup tangerine
4 tablespoons hulled
   hemp seed

Combine all ingredients in a high-power blender or food processor and blend until smooth. Drink immediately.

Serves 2

Nutrition Facts (per serving)

Calories 174
Fat 6 g
Carbs 25 g
Fiber 5 g
Protein 6 g

Jing K, Wu T, Lim K. (2013) Omega-3 polyunsaturated fatty acids and cancer. *Anti-Cancer Agents in Medicinal Chemistry*.

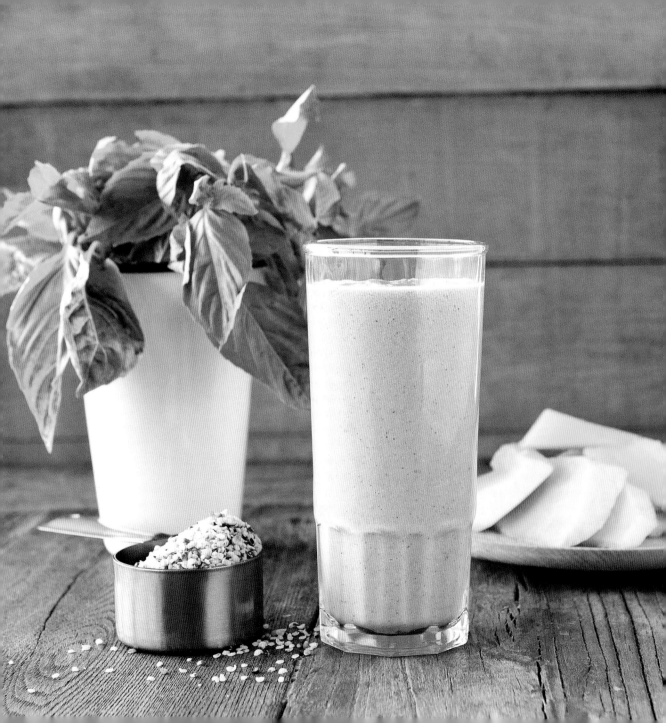

Sweet Basil Pom

Mangiferin is a polyphenol in mangos that has the ability to inhibit cancer cell growth by apoptosis.

Fresh basil and mango flavors predominate in this light, sweet combination.

Ingredients

1 cup frozen green tea cubes
½ cup pomegranate juice
½ cup frozen mango
½ cup fresh basil leaves
2 tablespoons hulled hemp seed

Combine all ingredients in a high-power blender or food processor and blend until smooth. Drink immediately.

Serves 2

Nutrition Facts (per serving)

Calories 112
Fat 3 g
Carbs 18 g
Fiber 2 g
Protein 3 g

Matkowski A, Kuś P, Góralska E, Woźniak D. (2013) Mangiferin – a bioactive xanthonoid, not only from mango and not just antioxidant. *Mini-Reviews in Medicinal Chemistry.*

Tea Cube Frosties

Tea leaves contain concentrated amounts of cancer-fighting nutrients that can be obtained through tisane (tea). The simple process of pouring hot water over tea leaves is what extracts these powerful nutrients. Once activated, the tea can then be ingested as hot tea, or chilled and consumed as cold tea, or frozen and added to drinks and smoothies.

Many types of tea leaves have been studied for their ability to reduce cancer cell growth. Black, green, white, and mint tea help reduce the risk for the development and recurrence of many types of cancer.

Green tea polyphenols such as epigallocatechin gallate (EGCG) have been found to instigate anti-neoplastic activity against cancer cells and provide protection from the development of various types of precancerous lesions by reducing cell growth and genetic damage. EGCG appears to be particularly effective in protecting against the development of breast and oral cancers.

Mint teas are of current interest in oncology nutrition as spearmint tea has been found to promote antimutagenic activity.

Pom Mango Berry

Green tea polyphenols exert a cancer-preventive effect against precancerous lesions by reducing cell growth and genetic damage.

This smoothie has robust berry and pomegranate flavors with undertones of mango and green tea.

Ingredients

½ cup pomegranate juice
½ cup frozen red
  raspberries
½ cup fresh mango
½ cup frozen green tea
  cubes
2 tablespoons chia seed

Combine all ingredients in a high-power blender or food processor and blend until smooth. Drink immediately.

Serves 2

Nutrition Facts (per serving)

Calories 167
Fat 6 g
Carbs 25 g
Fiber 11 g
Protein 4 g

Shen T, Khor SC, Zhou F, Duan T, Xu YY, Zheng YF, Hsu S, De Stefano J, Yang J, Xu LH, Zhu XQ. (2014) Chemoprevention by lipid-soluble tea polyphenols in diethylnitrosamine/phenobarbital-induced hepatic pre-cancerous lesions. *Anticancer Research*.

Phenolic Cooler

Tea (black, green, white, and spearmint) helps reduce the risk for the development and recurrence of many types of cancer.

This fresh summer fruit combination has sweet flavors balanced by refreshing green tea.

Ingredients
½ cup pomegranate juice
½ cup fresh watermelon
½ cup fresh pineapple
½ cup frozen red
  raspberries
½ cup frozen green tea
  cubes
2 tablespoons chia seed
1 teaspoon lemon juice

Combine all ingredients in a high-power blender or food processor and blend until smooth. Drink immediately.

Serves 2

Nutrition Facts (per serving)

Calories 208
Fat 5 g
Carbs 36 g
Fiber 10 g
Protein 4 g

Huang CC, et al. (2014) Tea consumption and risk of head and neck cancer. *PLoS One.*

EGCG Power

The green tea polyphenol known as epigallocatechin gallate (EGCG) has been found to have anti-neoplastic activity against cancer cells, particularly breast cancer cells.

This slightly sweet, fruity combination is light and refreshing and rich in protein.

Ingredients

1 cup frozen green tea cubes
½ cup pomegranate juice
½ cup watermelon
½ cup pineapple
2 tablespoons chia seed

Combine all ingredients in a high-power blender or food processor and blend until smooth. Drink immediately.

Serves 2

Nutrition Facts (per serving)

Calories 149
Fat 5 g
Carbs 21 g
Fiber 7 g
Protein 4 g

Manjegowda CM, Deb G, Limaye AM. (2014) Epigallocatechin gallate induces the steady state mRNA levels of pS2 and PR genes in MCF-7 breast cancer cells. *Indian Journal of Experimental Biology.*

Mango Melon Cherry

Watermelon is a rich source of lycopene, which has powerful antioxidant action against ovarian cancer cells in postmenopausal women.

This rich and creamy mango smoothie is satisfying and filling, yet light and fresh.

Ingredients

1 cup frozen green tea cubes
½ cup red tart cherry juice
½ cup watermelon
½ cup frozen mango
2 tablespoons hulled hemp seed

Combine all ingredients in a high-power blender or food processor and blend until smooth. Drink immediately.

Serves 2

Nutrition Facts (per serving)

Calories 129
Fat 3
Carbs 22 g
Fiber 2 g
Protein 4 g

Li-Xinli, Xu-Jiuhong. (2014) Meta-analysis of the association between dietary lycopene intake and ovarian cancer risk in postmenopausal women. *Scientific Reports.*

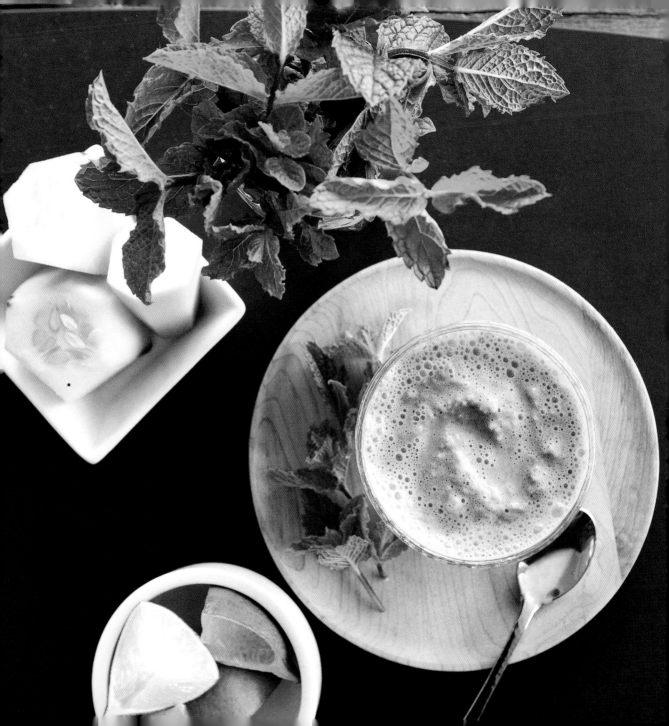

Cucumber Pom Mint

Cucurbitacin is a naturally occurring triterpenoid in cucumber that induces apoptosis (cancer cell destruction) and blocks the cell cycle progression of various cancers.

This light smoothie has fresh cucumber, mint, and pomegranate flavors.

Ingredients

1 lime wedge
½ cup frozen cucumber
½ cup frozen mint tea
   cubes
½ cup pomegranate juice
2 tablespoons hulled
   hemp seed

Combine all ingredients in a high-power blender or food processor and blend until smooth. Drink immediately.

Serves 1

Nutrition Facts (per serving)

Calories 169
Fat 6 g
Carbs 22 g
Fiber 4 g
Protein 6 g

Kim HJ, Kim JK. (2014) Antiangiogenic effects of cucurbitacin-I. *Archives of Pharmacology Research.*

Tart Peach Cream

Peaches contain numerous phytochemicals that protect against cancer by effecting signaling pathways that modulate cancer development.

This creamy peach and coconut smoothie has an edge of cranberry tartness.

Ingredients

½ cup cultured coconut milk
½ cup cranberry juice
½ cup frozen peaches
½ cup frozen green tea cubes
2 tablespoons chia seed

Combine all ingredients in a high-power blender or food processor and blend until smooth. Drink immediately.

Serves 1

Nutrition Facts (per serving)

Calories 250
Fat 13 g
Carb 26 g
Fiber 14 g
Protein 7 g

Yang MH, Kim J, Khan IA, Walker LA, Khan SI. (2014) Nonsteroidal anti-inflammatory drug activated gene-1 (NAG-1) modulators from natural products as anticancer agents. *Life Sciences*.

Vanilla Bean Cream

Vanilla contains vanillin and piperonal, which are compounds that arrest cancer cell growth and cause apoptosis of cancer cells.

Creamy, with fresh berry flavor, this smoothie has a potent vanilla bean fragrance.

Ingredients

1 vanilla bean
½ cup almond milk
¼ cup frozen strawberries
¼ cup frozen green tea cubes
2 tablespoons protein powder

Combine all ingredients in a high-power blender or food processor and blend until smooth. Drink immediately.

Serves 1

Nutrition Facts (per serving)

Calories 100
Fat 1 g
Carb 7 g
Fiber 1 g
Protein 13 g

Shi ZY, Li YQ, Kang YH, Hu GQ, Huang-fu CS, Deng JB, Liu B. (2012) Piperonal ciprofloxacin hydrazone induces growth arrest and apoptosis of human hepatocarcinoma SMMC-7721 cells. *Journal of the Chinese Pharmacological Society.*

Ginger Apple Berry

Spearmint possesses antimutagenic qualities that may provide protection against the development of cancer.

This smoothie has a spicy fragrance, with a spearmint base and subtle apple flavor.

Ingredients

1 cup spearmint tea
½ cup apple
½ cup frozen green tea cubes
½ cup frozen strawberries
¼ cup fresh basil leaves
2 tablespoons hulled hemp seed
1 tablespoon fresh ginger root
½ teaspoon cinnamon
¼ teaspoon cardamom

Combine all ingredients in a high-power blender or food processor and blend until smooth. Drink immediately.

Serves 2

Nutrition Facts (per serving)

Calories 73
Fat 3 g
Carbs 9 g
Fiber 3 g
Protein 3 g

Yu TW, Xu M, Dashwood RH. (2004) Antimutagenic activity of spearmint. *Environmental and Molecular Mutagenesis.*

Tropical Pom

Green tea has been found to provide protection from the development of various types of cancer, particularly breast and oral cancers.

This lush blend has subtle tea flavor while coconut and lime give this orange and berry smoothie a tropical fragrance.

Ingredients

1 lime wedge
½ cup frozen strawberries
½ cup frozen green tea
    cubes
½ cup pomegranate juice
½ cup orange juice
2 tablespoons shredded
    unsweetened coconut
2 tablespoons hulled
    hemp seed

Combine all ingredients in a high-power blender or food processor and blend until smooth. Drink immediately.

Serves 2

Nutrition Facts (per serving)

Calories 211
Fat 12 g
Carbs 22 g
Fiber 4 g
Protein 4 g

Wang W, Yang Y, Zhang W, Wu W. (2014) Association of tea consumption and the risk of oral cancer: a meta-analysis. *Oral Oncology.*

Cucumber Berry Mint

Cucumbers contain cucurbitacin, which is a natural antioxidant compound with anti-tumor properties as well as the ability to take potent preventive action against various types of cancer, including gliomas.

This tart and fresh smoothie tastes like a red Jolly Rancher candy. It has a fresh cucumber and light berry flavor, with lemon peel essence.

Ingredients

1 lemon wedge
½ cup frozen mint tea cubes
½ cup peeled, frozen cucumber
½ cup pomegranate juice
½ cup frozen strawberries
2 tablespoons hulled hemp seed

Combine all ingredients in a high-power blender or food processor and blend until smooth. Drink immediately.

Serves 2

Nutrition Facts (per serving)

Calories 96
Fat 3 g
Carbs 14 g
Fiber 2 g
Protein 3 g

Hsu YC, Chen MJ, Huang TY. (2014) Inducement of mitosis delay by cucurbitacin E, a novel tetracyclic triterpene from climbing stem of Cucumis melo L., through GADD45γ in human brain malignant glioma (GBM) 8401 cells. *Cell Death and Disease.*

Mint Currant

Melatonin, found in the whole fruit and juice of orange, pineapple, and banana, is an important antioxidant that interferes with the development of some cancers.

This pineapple and berry combination has a mint and green tea base with just a touch of tart cranberry.

Ingredients

½ cup mint tea
½ cup currant juice
½ cup pineapple
½ cup frozen strawberries
½ cup frozen green tea cubes
¼ cup cranberry
2 tablespoons hulled hemp seed

Combine all ingredients in a high-power blender or food processor and blend until smooth. Drink immediately.

Serves 2

Nutrition Facts (per serving)

Calories 100
Fat 3 g
Carbs 16 g
Fiber 3 g
Protein 3 g

Sae-Teaw M, Johns J, Johns NP, Subongkot S. (2013) Serum melatonin levels and antioxidant capacities after consumption of pineapple, orange, or banana by healthy male volunteers. *Journal of Pineal Research.*

Wild Blueberries

Wild blueberries are harvested in rugged natural terrain where the berries grow smaller, have richer flavor, and have extraordinarily high antioxidant levels. Wild blueberries contain concentrated amounts of the same health-promoting polyphenolic compounds as common blueberries.

These antioxidants protect against the oxidative cell damage and chronic inflammation that can lead to cancer. The antioxidant and anti-inflammatory action of wild berries have been well-studied for their potential to help prevent many diseases, including cancer.

The proanthocyanidins in wild blueberries are absorbed in our intestines when they are metabolized by the beneficial bacteria that line our gut wall. These organisms, such as acidophilus and bifidobacterium, can be added to smoothies in powder form or via cultured food products like cultured coconut milk.

Blueberry Pom Citrus

Wild blueberries contain antioxidants that reduce the chronic inflammation that causes the oxidative cell damage, which can lead to cancer.

This smoothie has layers of berry, citrus, and tea flavors and is rich in anthocyanins.

Ingredients

1 cup frozen green tea cubes
½ cup frozen wild blueberries
½ cup pomegranate seeds
½ cup orange juice
2 tablespoons protein powder

Combine all ingredients in a high-power blender or food processor and blend until smooth. Drink immediately.

Serves 2

Nutrition Facts (per serving)

Calories 121
Fat 0 g
Carbs 23 g
Fiber 4 g
Protein 7 g

Dinstel RR, Cascio J, Koukel S. (2013) The antioxidant level of Alaska's wild berries: high, higher and highest. *International Journal of Circumpolar Health.*

Wild Blueberry and Currant

Blueberry nutrients have an epigenetic effect on the development of cancer in humans by reducing oxidative damage to DNA.

This wild blueberry and currant juice smoothie with lemon essence is refreshing and light.

Ingredients

1 lemon wedge
1 cup frozen wild
   blueberries
½ cup currant juice
½ cup carrot juice
½ cup frozen green tea
   cubes
2 tablespoons chia seed

Combine all ingredients in a high-power blender or food processor and blend until smooth. Drink immediately.

Serves 2

Nutrition Facts (per serving)

Calories 138
Fat 5 g
Carbs 17 g
Fiber 6 g
Protein 4 g

Wilms LC, Boots AW, de Boer VC, Maas LM, Pachen DM, Gottschalk RW, Ketelslegers HB, Godschalk RW, Haenen GR, van Schooten FJ, Kleinjans JC. (2007) Impact of multiple genetic polymorphisms on effects of a 4-week blueberry juice intervention on ex vivo induced lymphocytic DNA damage in human volunteers. *Carcinogenesis.*

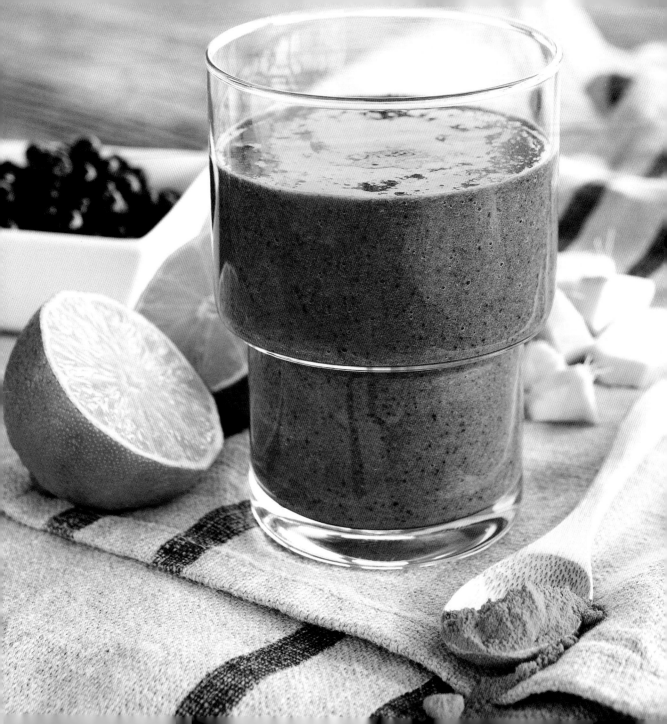

The Elysemo

Red blood oranges contain flavonoids, carotenoids, ascorbic acid, hydroxycinnamic acids, and anthocyanins that efficiently counteract the oxidative damage that plays a role in the development of cancer.

This smoothie is a rich blend of crushed citrus flavors and herbal fragrance.

Ingredients

1 cup blood orange
½ cup Meyer's lemon
½ cup lime
½ cup frozen wild
   blueberries
2 tablespoons protein
   powder
1 tablespoon fresh ginger
   root
½ teaspoon turmeric
   powder

Combine all ingredients in a high-power blender or food processor and blend until smooth. Drink immediately.

Serves 2

Nutrition Facts (per serving)

Calories 170
Fat 0 g
Carbs 42 g
Fiber 10 g
Protein 8 g

Grosso G, Galvano F, Mistretta A, Marventano S, Nolfo F, Calabrese G, Buscemi S, Drago F, Veronesi U, Scuderi A. (2013) Red orange: experimental models and epidemiological evidence of its benefits on human health. *Oxidative Medicine and Cellular Longevity*.

Cherry Citrus Rosemary

Rosemary contains betulinic and carnosic acids which have antioxidant, cytotoxic, and immunomodifying effects against cancer development.

This combination has intense fruit flavor balanced with complex herbal accents.

Ingredients

½ cup blood orange
½ cup tart cherry juice
½ cup frozen green tea
   cubes
½ cup frozen wild
   blueberries
2 tablespoons chia seed
1 tablespoon fresh
   rosemary

Combine all ingredients in a high-power blender or food processor and blend until smooth. Drink immediately.

Serves 2

Nutrition Facts (per serving)

Calories 157
Fat 5 g
Carbs 23 g
Fiber 9 g
Protein 4 g

Kontogianni VG, Tomic G, Nikolic I, Nerantzaki AA, Sayyad N, Stosic-Grujicic S, Stojanovic I, Gerothanassis IP, Tzakos AG. (2013) Phytochemical profile of Rosmarinus officinalis and Salvia officinalis extracts and correlation to their antioxidant and antiproliferative activity. *Food Chemistry.*

Catechin Elixir

Apple skins contain the nutrients catechins, flavonols, and quercetin, which have been found to regulate cell invasion, metastasis, and angiogenesis.

This frosty apple and wild blueberry combination is a little spicy from the ginger and the pepper.

Ingredients

½ cup currant juice
½ cup apple
½ cup wild blueberries
½ cup frozen green tea cubes
¼ cup carrot juice
2 tablespoons hulled hemp seed
1 tablespoon fresh ginger root
½ teaspoon turmeric powder
¼ teaspoon black pepper

Combine all ingredients in a high-power blender or food processor and blend until smooth. Drink immediately.

Serves 2

Nutrition Facts (per serving)

Calories 94
Fat 3 g
Carbs 14 g
Fiber 2 g
Protein 3 g

Reagan-Shaw S, Eggert D, Mukhtar H, Ahmad N. (2010) Antiproliferative effects of apple peel extract against cancer cells. *Nutrition and Cancer.*

Berry and Rosemary Healer

Rosemary contains a medicinal compound called carnosol that directly reduces cancer growth and development.

This berry and herbal smoothie is a perfectly balanced blend of sweet, sour, and bitter.

Ingredients

1 cup orange juice
½ cup pomegranate seeds
½ cup frozen wild
  blueberries
½ cup frozen blackberries
2 tablespoons chia seed
1 tablespoon fresh
  rosemary

Combine all ingredients in a high-power blender or food processor and blend until smooth. Drink immediately.

Serves 2

Nutrition Facts (per serving)

Calories 187
Fat 5 g
Carbs 29 g
Fiber 13 g
Protein 5 g

Khuda-Bukhsh AR, Das S, Saha SK. (2014) Molecular approaches toward targeted cancer prevention with some food plants and their products: inflammatory and other signal pathways. *Nutrition and Cancer.*

Quercetin Thirst Quencher

Natural antioxidant compounds in apples, which include procyanidins, catechins, flavonols, and quercetin, exert chemopreventive properties via cell cycle control.

This light smoothie is fresh and frosty with sweet carrot flavor and an herbal tea fragrance.

Ingredients

½ cup carrot juice
½ cup frozen wild
   blueberries
½ cup apple
½ cup frozen green tea
   cubes
2 tablespoons chia seed

Combine all ingredients in a high-power blender or food processor and blend until smooth. Drink immediately.

Serves 2

Nutrition Facts (per serving)

Calories 132
Fat 5 g
Carbs 17 g
Fiber 10 g
Protein 3 g

Ribeiro FA, Gomes de Moura CF, Aguiar O Jr, de Oliveira F, Spadari RC, Oliveira NR, Oshima CT, Ribeiro DA. (2013) The chemopreventive activity of apple against carcinogenesis: antioxidant activity and cell cycle control. *European Journal of Cancer Prevention.*

Berry Sorbet

Carnosol, an active constituent of rosemary, is an anti–inflammatory agent that has the ability to trigger apoptosis.

The intense flavor and fragrant rosemary and berry scents in this smoothie create a sorbet-like experience.

Ingredients

½ cup orange juice
½ cup frozen wild
  blueberries
½ cup frozen green tea
  cubes
2 tablespoons chia seed
1 tablespoon fresh
  rosemary

Combine all ingredients in a high-power blender or food processor and blend until smooth. Drink immediately.

Serves 1

Nutrition Facts (per serving)

Calories 253
Fat 10 g
Carbs 31 g
Fiber 17 g
Protein 7 g

Park KW, Kundu J, Chae IG, Kim DH, Yu MH, Kundu JK, Chun KS. (2014) Carnosol induces apoptosis through generation of ROS and inactivation of STAT3 signaling in human colon cancer HCT116 cells. *International Journal of Oncology*.

The Blue Cranberry

Anthocyanins from blueberries have been shown to encourage anticancer activity by reducing oxidative damage throughout the body and at specific cancer sites.

This wild blueberry smoothie is rich in berry flavor with a balance of sweet watermelon and tart cranberry.

Ingredients

½ cup wild blueberries
½ cup watermelon
½ cup frozen green tea
  cubes
¼ cup cranberry juice
2 tablespoons chia seed

Combine all ingredients in a high-power blender or food processor and blend until smooth. Drink immediately.

Serves 1

Nutrition Facts (per serving)

Calories 262
Fat 10 g
Carbs 35 g
Fiber 18 g
Protein 7 g

Aqil F, Vadhanam MV, Jeyabalan J, Cai J, Singh IP, Gupta RC. (2014) Detection of Anthocyanins/Anthocyanidins in Animal Tissues. *Journal of Agricultural Food Chemistry.*

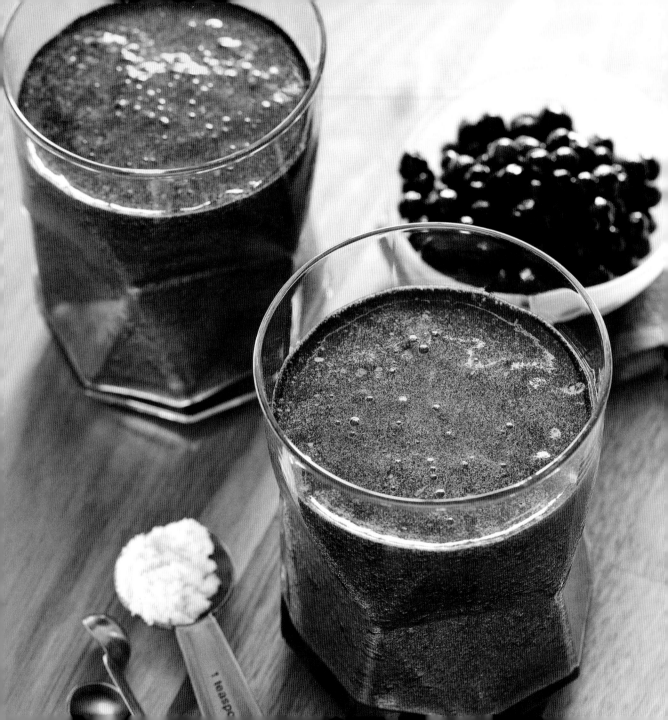

Black Currant and Wild Blueberry

Blueberries are rich in phenolic compounds, which are high in antioxidants and thus inhibit the production of pro-inflammatory molecules, reduce oxidative stress, lessen DNA damage, and thwart cancer cell proliferation overall.

This smoothie has sweet wild blueberry and rich currant berry color and flavor.

Ingredients

½ cup frozen wild
    blueberries
½ cup black currant juice
½ cup frozen green tea
    cubes
2 tablespoons protein
    powder

Combine all ingredients in a high-power blender or food processor and blend until smooth. Drink immediately.

Serves 1

Nutrition Facts (per serving)

Calories 108
Fat 0 g
Carbs 12 g
Fiber 0 g
Protein 13 g

Johnson SA, Arjmandi BH. (2013) Evidence for anticancer properties of blueberries: a mini-review. *Anticancer Agents in Medicinal Chemistry.*

Medical Terms

Medical terminology is included to help accurately convey the well-studied activity of the specific food nutrients I've used. Most medical definitions can be found on Wikipedia and a few of the most commonly used terms in the book are defined below.

Anticancer
A food, medication, or treatment that is termed "anticancer" is one that fights cancer whether by selective destruction of cancer cells or by enhancing an organism's natural defenses against cancer.

Angiogenesis
Angiogenesis is the growth of new blood vessels from pre-existing blood vessels. These vessels supply cells or benign (harmless) tumors with blood and nutrients for growth, although the tumor may then become malignant (cancerous).

Anti-inflammatory
Anti- (against) and inflammatory (inflammation-causing) is a term used for a substance such as a food, nutrient, or medication that reduces inflammation.

Antimutagenic
A mutagen is a physical or chemical agent that changes or damages genetic material, which can lead to cancer. Nutrients that reduce mutagenic activity are considered antimutagenic.

Antioxidant

Any molecule that inhibits oxidation of other molecules is an antioxidant. Many nutrients act as antioxidants, reducing free radicals and thus the risk for oxidative damage to cells and tissues.

Antiproliferative

This term is used to describe the reduction of growth and spread of cancer cells.

Apoptosis

Apoptosis is the process of programmed cell death that our bodies use to remove unhealthy or damaged cells. This system is very efficient and causes a cell to break up so that white blood cells can engulf the small pieces and remove them completely.

Apoptosis is a normal healthy function of the body. In fact, about sixty billion cells die each day in the average adult due to apoptosis. It's the body's way of cleaning up cancer cells and other cells that have formed incorrectly so that they do not divide and continue producing more abnormal cells.

Autophagy

Cell degradation by self-destruction is called autophagy. Food nutrients can trigger autophagy; for example, pineapple, which contains an enzyme called bromelain, has been shown to trigger autophagy of breast cancer cells.

Benign

This term generally refers to tumors that are harmless, slow growing, and not malignant.

Bioactive

This term has traditionally been applied to pharmacological activity but it can also be used to describe the effects of a nutrient or toxin on living matter. Biological activity describes either the beneficial or adverse effects of a substance on living matter.

Bioavailable
This term refers to the level of absorption of nutrients and medication.

Epigenetics
The study of genetics and triggers for genetic expression is termed epigenetics and includes environmental toxins, nutrients, hormones and many internal and external factors.

GMO
A genetically modified organism, which can be any living thing. For example, a plant, animal, or bacteria is called a GMO when its genetic material has been altered in a laboratory, not to be confused with natural genetic alternations such as crossbreeding.

Hormone Sensitive
Some tumors are made up of cells with specific hormone receptors. For example, if the cells react to estrogen, they are termed ER+ (Estrogen Receptor Positive), or PR+ (Progesterone Receptor Positive). If they do not respond to these hormones they are termed accordingly such as ER- (Estrogen Receptor Negative). Cells that are hormone sensitive depend on hormones for stimulation and growth.

Hyperplasia
The increase in the number of cells, which can lead to enlargement of organs, is hyperplasia.

Immunomodulating
Internal and external factors can change the way the immune system responds to invasion as in the case of cancer. Food nutrients, medical treatment, physical treatments, emotional states, and environmental toxins are all examples of factors that can affect the immune system's ability to function.

Metastasis
The spread of cancer from one organ to another is metastasis.

Microbiome
The microbiome is a term used to encompass the symbiotic and pathogenic microorganisms that live in and on our bodies.

Oligosaccharides
Dietary oligosaccharides such as fructo-oligosaccharides are molecules made of a group of simple sugars found in vegetables and fruit that are not completely digestible. They act as prebiotics, which are food for the healthy bacteria in our digestive tracts.

Phthalates
Compounds in plastics called phthalates have been found to stimulate cancer cell growth. Phthalates such as BPA are often in plastic food storage containers and are therefore of concern.

Prebiotics
Indigestible fiber becomes "prebiotic" once it reaches the large intestine on its way through the digestive tract. There it acts as food for the flora of the gut, helping to stimulate the growth and activity of these healthful bacteria.

Probiotics
Probiotics are the microorganisms (healthy bacteria) ingested either as a supplement or via cultured foods such as yogurt, kimchee, or sauerkraut.

Recurrence
A relapse of a condition that had been in remission is considered a recurrence.

References

ALMOND MILK
Tate PL, Bibb R, Larcom LL. (2011) Milk stimulates growth of prostate cancer cells in culture. *Nutrition and Cancer.*

APPLES
Reagan-Shaw S, Eggert D, Mukhtar H, Ahmad N. (2010) Antiproliferative effects of apple peel extract against cancer cells. *Nutrition and Cancer.*

Ribeiro FA, Gomes de Moura CF, Aguiar O Jr, de Oliveira F, Spadari RC, Oliveira NR, Oshima CT, Ribeiro DA. (2013) The chemopreventive activity of apple against carcinogenesis: antioxidant activity and cell cycle control. *European Journal of Cancer Prevention.*

BANANA
Bennett RN, Shiga TM, Hassimotto NM, Rosa EA, Lajolo FM, Cordenunsi BR. (2010) Phenolics and antioxidant properties of fruit pulp and cell wall fractions of postharvest banana (Musa acuminata Juss.) cultivars. *Journal of Agricultural and Food Chemistry.*

Kanazawa K, Sakakibara H. (2000) High content of dopamine, a strong antioxidant, in Cavendish banana. *Journal of Agricultural and Food Chemistry.*

Sae-Teaw M, Johns J, Johns NP, Subongkot S. (2012) Serum melatonin levels and antioxidant capacities after consumption of pineapple, orange, or banana by healthy male volunteers. *Journal of Pineal Research.*

Slavin J. (2013) Fiber and prebiotics: mechanisms and health benefits. *Nutrients.*

BASIL
Al-Ali KH, El-Beshbishy HA, El-Badry AA, Alkhalaf M. (2013) Cytotoxic activity of methanolic extract of Mentha longifolia and Ocimum basilicum against human breast cancer. *Pakistan Journal of Biological Sciences.*

Lv J, Shao Q, Wang H, Shi H, Wang T, Gao W, Song B, Zheng G, Kong B, Qu X. (2013) Effects and mechanisms of curcumin and basil polysaccharide on the invasion of SKOV3 cells and dendritic cells. *Molecular Medicine Reports.*

BLACKBERRIES
Seeram, NP. (2006) Blackberry, black raspberry, blueberry, cranberry, red raspberry, and strawberry extracts inhibit growth and stimulate apoptosis of human cancer cells in vitro. *Journal of Agricultural and Food Chemistry.*

BLACK PEPPER
Doucette CD, Hilchie AL, Liwski R, Hoskin DW. (2012) Piperine, a dietary phytochemical, inhibits angiogenesis. *The Journal of Nutritional Biochemistry.*

Majdalawieh, AF, & Carr, RI. (2010). In Vitro Investigation of the Potential Immunomodulatory and Anticancer Activities of Black Pepper (Piper nigrum) and Cardamom (Elettaria cardamomum). *Journal of Medicinal Food.*

BLOOD ORANGE
Grosso G, Galvano F, Mistretta A, Marventano S, Nolfo F, Calabrese G, Buscemi S, Drago F, Veronesi U, Scuderi A. (2013) Red orange: experimental models and epidemiological evidence of its benefits on human health. *Oxidative Medicine and Cellular Longevity.*

BLUEBERRIES
Aqil F, Vadhanam MV, Jeyabalan J, Cai J, Singh IP, Gupta RC. (2014) Detection of Anthocyanins/Anthocyanidins in Animal Tissues. *Journal of Agricultural Food Chemistry.*

Johnson SA, Arjmandi BH. (2013) Evidence for anticancer properties of blueberries: a mini-review. *Anticancer Agents in Medicinal Chemistry*.

Qureshi SA, Lund AC, Veierød MB, Carlsen MH, Blomhoff R, Andersen LF, Ursin G. (2014) Food items contributing most to variation in antioxidant intake; a cross-sectional study among Norwegian women. *BMC Public Health*.

Seeram, NP. (2006) Blackberry, black raspberry, blueberry, cranberry, red raspberry, and strawberry extracts inhibit growth and stimulate apoptosis of human cancer cells in vitro. *Journal of Agricultural and Food Chemistry*.

Wilms LC, Boots AW, de Boer VC, Maas LM, Pachen DM, Gottschalk RW, Ketelslegers HB, Godschalk RW, Haenen GR, van Schooten FJ, Kleinjans JC. (2007) Impact of multiple genetic polymorphisms on effects of a 4-week blueberry juice intervention on ex vivo induced lymphocytic DNA damage in human volunteers. *Carcinogenesis*.

CARDAMOM
Acharya A, Das I, Singh S, Saha T. (2010) Chemopreventive properties of indole-3-carbinol, diindolylmethane and other constituents of cardamom against carcinogenesis. *Recent Patents of Food, Nutrition and Agriculture*.

Majdalawieh, AF, & Carr, RI. (2010). In Vitro Investigation of the Potential Immunomodulatory and Anticancer Activities of Black Pepper (Piper nigrum) and Cardamom (Elettaria cardamomum). *Journal of Medicinal Food*.

CARROT
Butalla AC, Crane TE, Patil B, Wertheim BC, Thompson P, Thomson CA. (2012) Effects of a carrot juice intervention on plasma carotenoids, oxidative stress, and inflammation in overweight breast cancer survivors. *Nutrition and Cancer*.

Xu X, Cheng Y, Li S, Zhu Y, Xu X, Zheng X, Mao Q, Xie L. (2014) Dietary carrot consumption and the risk of prostate cancer. *European Journal of Nutrition*.

CAYENNE
Anandakumar P, Kamaraj S, Jagan S, Ramakrishnan G, Devaki T. (2013) Capsaicin provokes apoptosis and restricts benzo(a)pyrene induced lung tumorigenesis in Swiss albino mice. *International Immunopharmacology*.

CHERRIES
Khoo GM, Clausen MR, Pedersen BH, Larsen E. (2012) Bioactivity of sour cherry cultivars grown in Denmark. *Phytotherapy Research*.

Olsson, ME. (2004). Inhibition of cancer cell proliferation in vitro by fruit and berry extracts and correlations with antioxidant levels. *Journal of Agricultural and Food Chemistry*.

McCune LM, Kubota C, Stendell-Hollis NR, Thomson CA. (2011) Cherries and health: a review. *Critical Reviews in Food Science Nutrition*.

CHIA SEED
Ulbricht C, Chao W, Nummy K, Rusie E, Tanguay-Colucci S, Iannuzzi CM, Plammoottil JB, Varghese M, Weissner W. (2009) Chia (Salvia hispanica): a systematic review by the natural standard research collaboration. *Reviews on Recent Clinical Trials*.

Kurihara T, Kawamoto J. (2014) Chemical approach to analyze the physiological function of phospholipids with polyunsaturated Fatty acyl chain. *Yakugaku Zasshi*.

CITRUS
Baek SH, Kim SM, Nam D, Lee JH, Ahn KS, Choi SH, Kim SH, Shim BS, Chang IM, Ahn KS. (2012) Antimetastatic effect of nobiletin through the down-

regulation of CXC chemokine receptor type 4 and matrix metallopeptidase-9. *Pharmaceutical Biology.*

Bharti S, Rani N, Krishnamurthy B, Arya DS. (2014) Preclinical Evidence for the Pharmacological Actions of Naringin: A Review. *Planta Medica.*

Dong Y, Cao A, Shi J, Yin P, Wang L, Ji G, Xie J, Wu D. (2014) Tangeretin, a citrus polymethoxy flavonoid, induces apoptosis of human gastric cancer AGS cells through extrinsic and intrinsic signaling pathways. *Oncology Reports.*

Tanaka T, Tanaka T, Tanaka M, Kuno T. (2011) Cancer chemoprevention by citrus pulp and juices containing high amounts of β-cryptoxanthin and hesperidin. *BioMed Research International.*

COCOA
Fernandes I, Marques F, de Freitas V, Mateus N. (2013) Antioxidant and antiproliferative properties of methylated metabolites of anthocyanins. *Food Chemistry.*

Kim J, Shim J, Lee CY, Lee KW, Lee HJ. (2014) Cocoa phytochemicals: recent advances in molecular mechanisms on health. *Critical Reviews in Food Science and Nutrition.*

Sugimoto N, Miwa S, Hitomi Y, Nakamura H, Tsuchiya H, Yachie A. (2014) Theobromine, the Primary Methylxanthine Found in Theobroma cacao, Prevents Malignant Glioblastoma Proliferation by Negatively Regulating Phosphodiesterase-4, Extracellular Signal-regulated Kinase, Akt/mammalian Target of Rapamycin Kinase, and Nuclear Factor-Kappa B. *Nutrition and Cancer.*

CRANBERRIES
Katsargyris A, Tampaki EC, Giaginis C, Theocharis S. (2012) Cranberry as promising natural source of potential anticancer agents: current evidence and future perspectives. *Anticancer Agents Medicinal Chemistry*.

Khuda-Bukhsh AR, Das S, Saha SK. (2014) Molecular approaches toward targeted cancer prevention with some food plants and their products: inflammatory and other signal pathways. *Nutrition and Cancer*.

CREATINE
de Campos-Ferraz PL, Andrade I, das Neves W, Hangai I, Alves CR, Lancha Jr AH. (2014) An overview of amines as nutritional supplements to counteract cancer cachexia. *Journal of Cachexia, Sarcopenia and Muscle*.

CUCUMBER
Gao Y, Islam MS, Tian J, Lui VW, Xiao D. (2014) Inactivation of ATP citrate lyase by Cucurbitacin B: A bioactive compound from cucumber, inhibits prostate cancer growth. *Cancer Letters*.

Hsu YC, Chen MJ, Huang TY. (2014) Inducement of mitosis delay by cucurbitacin E, a novel tetracyclic triterpene from climbing stem of Cucumis melo L., through GADD45γ in human brain malignant glioma (GBM) 8401 cells. *Cell Death and Disease*.

Kim HJ, Kim JK. (2014) Antiangiogenic effects of cucurbitacin-I. *Archives of Pharmacal Research*.

CULTURED COCONUT MILK
Tarko T, Duda-Chodak A, Zajac N. (2013) Digestion and absorption of phenolic compounds assessed by in vitro simulation methods. *Annals of the National Institute of Hygiene*.

Walsh CJ, Guinane CM, O'Toole PW, Cotter PD. (2014) Beneficial modulation of the gut microbiota. *Federation of European Biochemical Societies Letters.*

Ewaschuk JB, Walker JW, Diaz H, Madsen KL. (2006) Bioproduction of conjugated linoleic acid by probiotic bacteria occurs in vitro and in vivo in mice. *Journal of Nutrition.*

CURRANTS
Erlund I, Freese R, Marniemi J, Hakala P, Alfthan G. Bioavailability of quercetin from berries and the diet. (2006) *Nutrition and Cancer.*

GARLIC
Chandra-Kuntal K, Lee J, Singh SV. (2013) Critical role for reactive oxygen species in apoptosis induction and cell migration inhibition by diallyl trisulfide, a cancer chemopreventive component of garlic. *Breast Cancer Treatment and Research.*

Chu YL, Raghu R, Lu KH, Liu CT, Lin SH, Lai YS, Cheng WC, Lin SH, Sheen LY. (2013) Autophagy Therapeutic Potential of Garlic in Human Cancer Therapy. *Journal of Traditional Complementary Medicine.*

Galeone C. (2006) Onion and garlic use and human cancer. *American Journal of Clinical Nutrition.*

Ma HB, Huang S, Yin XR, Zhang Y, Di ZL. (2014) Apoptotic pathway induced by diallyl trisulfide in pancreatic cancer cells. *World Journal of Gastroenterology.*

Milner, John A. (2006) Preclinical Perspectives on Garlic and Cancer. *The Journal of Nutrition.*

Khuda-Bukhsh AR, Das S, Saha SK. (2014) Molecular approaches toward targeted cancer prevention with some food plants and their products: inflammatory and other signal pathways. *Nutrition and Cancer.*

Yun HM, Ban JO, Park KR, Lee CK, Jeong HS, Han SB, Hong JT. (2014) Potential therapeutic effects of functionally active compounds isolated from garlic. *Pharmacology & Therapeutics*.

GINGER
Gan FF, Ling H, Ang X, Reddy SA, Lee SS, Yang H, Tan SH, Hayes JD, Chui WK, Chew EH. (2013) A novel shogaol analog suppresses cancer cell invasion and inflammation, and displays cytoprotective effects through modulation of NF-κB and Nrf2-Keap1 signaling pathways. *Toxicology and Applied Pharmacology*.

Poltronieri J, Becceneri AB, Fuzer AM, C Filho JC, B M Martin AC, Vieira PC, Pouliot N, Cominetti MR. (2014) [6]-gingerol as a Cancer Chemopreventive Agent: A Review of Its Activity on Different Steps of the Metastatic Process. *Mini-Reviews in Medicinal Chemistry*.

Sultan MT, Butt MS, Qayyum MM, Suleria HA. (2014) Immunity: plants as effective mediators. *Critical Reviews in Food Science and Nutrition*.

GRAPES
Gambini J, López-Grueso R, Olaso-González G, Inglés M, Abdelazid K, El Alami M, Bonet-Costa V, Borrás C, Viña J. (2013) Resveratrol: distribution, properties and perspectives. *Review Spanish Geriatrics & Gerontology*.

Khuda-Bukhsh AR1, Das S, Saha SK. (2014) Molecular approaches toward targeted cancer prevention with some food plants and their products: inflammatory and other signal pathways. *Nutrition and Cancer*.

Xue YQ, Di JM, Luo Y, Cheng KJ, Wei X, Shi Z. (2014) Resveratrol Oligomers for the Prevention and Treatment of Cancers. *Oxidative Medicine Cellular Longevity Journal*.

GRAPEFRUIT
Baek SH, Kim SM, Nam D, Lee JH, Ahn KS, Choi SH, Kim SH, Shim BS, Chang IM, Ahn KS. (2012) Antimetastatic effect of nobiletin through the down-regulation of CXC chemokine receptor type 4 and matrix metallopeptidase-9. *Pharmaceutical Biology.*

Bhuvaneswari V, & Nagini S. (2005) Lycopene: a review of its potential as an anticancer agent. *Current Medicinal Therapy—Anti-Cancer Agents.*

Tong LX, Young LC. (2014) Nutrition: The future of melanoma prevention? *Journal of the American Academy of Dermatology.*

Lin CW, Chen PN, Chen MK, Yang WE, Tang CH, Yang SF, Hsieh YS. (2013) Kaempferol reduces matrix metalloproteinase-2 expression by down-regulating ERK1/2 and the activator protein-1 signaling pathways in oral cancer cells. *PLoS One.*

Yu L, Chen C, Wang LF, Kuang X, Liu K, Zhang H, Du JR. (2013) Neuroprotective effect of kaempferol glycosides against brain injury and neuroinflammation by inhibiting the activation of NF-κB and STAT3 in transient focal stroke. *PLoS One.*

Kong L, Luo C, Li X, Zhou Y, He H. (2013) The anti-inflammatory effect of kaempferol on early atherosclerosis in high cholesterol fed rabbits. *Lipids in Health and Disease.*

GREEN TEA
Onakpoya I, Spencer E, Heneghan C, Thompson M. (2014) The effect of green tea on blood pressure and lipid profile: A systematic review and meta-analysis of randomized clinical trials. *Nutrition Metabolism and Cardiovascular Disease.*

Donejko M, Niczyporuk M, Galicka E, Przylipiak A. (2013) Anticancer properties epigallocatechin-gallate contained in green tea. *Postepy Hig Med Dosw.*

Shen T, Khor SC, Zhou F, Duan T, Xu YY, Zheng YF, Hsu S, De Stefano J, Yang J, Xu LH, Zhu XQ. (2014) Chemoprevention by lipid-soluble tea polyphenols in diethylnitrosamine/phenobarbital-induced hepatic precancerous lesions. *Anticancer Research.*

Manjegowda CM, Deb G, Limaye AM. (2014) Epigallocatechin gallate induces the steady state mRNA levels of pS2 and PR genes in MCF-7 breast cancer cells. *Indian Journal of Experimental Biology.*

HEMP SEED

Notarnicola M, Tutino V, Caruso MG. (2014) Tumor-Induced Alterations in Lipid Metabolism. *Current Medicinal Chemistry.*

Jing K, Wu T, Lim K. (2013) Omega-3 polyunsaturated fatty acids and cancer. *Anti-Cancer Agents in Medicinal Chemistry.*

HOLY BASIL

Baliga MS, Jimmy R, Thilakchand KR, Sunitha V, Bhat NR, Saldanha E, Rao S, Rao P, Arora R, Palatty PL. (2013) Ocimum sanctum L (Holy Basil or Tulsi) and its phytochemicals in the prevention and treatment of cancer. *Nutrition and Cancer.*

Bhattacharyya P, Bishayee A. (2013) Ocimum sanctum Linn. (Tulsi): an ethnomedicinal plant for the prevention and treatment of cancer. *Anticancer Drugs.*

Shimizu T, Torres MP, Chakraborty S, Souchek JJ, Rachagani S, Kaur S, Macha M, Ganti AK, Hauke RJ, Batra SK. (2013) Holy Basil leaf extract decreases tumorigenicity and metastasis of aggressive human pancreatic cancer cells in vitro and in vivo: potential role in therapy. *Cancer Letters.*

KUMQUAT
Tundis R, Loizzo MR, Menichini F. (2014) An overview on chemical aspects and potential health benefits of limonoids and their derivatives. *Critical Reviews in Food Science and Nutrition.*

LEMON
Baek SH, Kim SM, Nam D, Lee JH, Ahn KS, Choi SH, Kim SH, Shim BS, Chang IM, Ahn KS. (2012) Antimetastatic effect of nobiletin through the down-regulation of CXC chemokine receptor type 4 and matrix metallopeptidase-9. *Pharmaceutical Biology.*

Dong Y, Cao A, Shi J, Yin P, Wang L, Ji G, Xie J, Wu D. (2014) Tangeretin, a citrus polymethoxy flavonoid, induces apoptosis of human gastric cancer AGS cells through extrinsic and intrinsic signaling pathways. *Oncology Reports.*

Lakshmi A, Subramanian S. (2014) Chemotherapeutic effect of tangeretin, a polymethoxylated flavone studied in 7, 12-dimethylbenz(a)anthracene induced mammary carcinoma in experimental rats. *Biochimie.*

Tundis R, Loizzo MR, Menichini F. (2014) An overview on chemical aspects and potential health benefits of limonoids and their derivatives. *Critical Reviews in Food Science and Nutrition.*

LIME
Lakshmi A, Subramanian S. (2014) Chemotherapeutic effect of tangeretin, a polymethoxylated flavone studied in 7, 12-dimethylbenz(a)anthracene induced mammary carcinoma in experimental rats. *Biochimie.*

Tundis R, Loizzo MR, Menichini F. (2014) An overview on chemical aspects and potential health benefits of limonoids and their derivatives. *Critical Reviews in Food Science and Nutrition.*

Charles C, Nachtergael A, Ouedraogo M, Belayew A, Duez P. (2014) Effects of chemopreventive natural products on non-homologous end-joining DNA double-strand break repair. *Mutation Research*.

MANDARIN ORANGE
Lakshmi A, Subramanian S. (2014) Chemotherapeutic effect of tangeretin, a polymethoxylated flavone studied in 7, 12-dimethylbenz(a)anthracene induced mammary carcinoma in experimental rats. *Biochimie*.

Wu C, Han L, Riaz H, Wang S, Cai K, Yang L. (2013) The chemopreventive effect of β-cryptoxanthin from mandarin on human stomach cells (BGC-823). *Food Chemistry*.

MANGO
Matkowski A, Kuś P, Góralska E, Woźniak D. (2013) Mangiferin - a bioactive xanthonoid, not only from mango and not just antioxidant. *Mini-Reviews in Medicinal Chemistry*.

Wilkinson AS, Flanagan BM, Pierson JT, Hewavitharana AK, Dietzgen RG, Shaw PN, Roberts-Thomson SJ, Monteith GR, Gidley MJ. (2011) Bioactivity of mango flesh and peel extracts on peroxisome proliferator-activated receptor γ [PPARγ] activation and MCF-7 cell proliferation: fraction and fruit variability. *Journal of Food Science*.

ORANGES
Baek SH, Kim SM, Nam D, Lee JH, Ahn KS, Choi SH, Kim SH, Shim BS, Chang IM, Ahn KS. (2012) Antimetastatic effect of nobiletin through the down-regulation of CXC chemokine receptor type 4 and matrix metallopeptidase-9. *Pharmaceutical Biology*.

Lakshmi A, Subramanian S. (2014) Chemotherapeutic effect of tangeretin, a polymethoxylated flavone studied in 7, 12-dimethylbenz(a)anthracene induced mammary carcinoma in experimental rats. *Biochimie*.

Sae-Teaw M, Johns J, Johns NP, Subongkot S. (2013) Serum melatonin levels and antioxidant capacities after consumption of pineapple, orange, or banana by healthy male volunteers. *Journal of Pineal Research.*

Tundis R, Loizzo MR, Menichini F. (2014) An overview on chemical aspects and potential health benefits of limonoids and their derivatives. *Critical Reviews in Food Science and Nutrition.*

PAPAYA
Nguyen TT, Shaw PN, Parat MO, Hewavitharana AK. (2013). Anticancer activity of Carica papaya: a review. *Molecular Nutrition & Food Research.*

Li ZY, Wang Y, Shen WT, Zhou P. (2012) Content determination of benzyl glucosinolate and anticancer activity of its hydrolysis product in Carica papaya L. *Asian Pacific Journal of Tropical Medicine.*

PEACHES
Yang MH, Kim J, Khan IA, Walker LA, Khan SI. (2014) Nonsteroidal anti-inflammatory drug activated gene-1 (NAG-1) modulators from natural products as anticancer agents. *Life Sciences.*

PEANUTS
Altamemi I, Murphy EA, Catroppo JF, Zumbrun EE, Zhang J, McClellan JL, Singh UP, Nagarkatti PS, Nagarkatti M. (2014) Role of microRNAs in resveratrol-mediated mitigation of colitis-associated tumorigenesis in ApcMin/+ mice. *Journal of Pharmacology and Experimental Therapeutics.*

Khuda-Bukhsh AR, Das S, Saha SK. (2014) Molecular approaches toward targeted cancer prevention with some food plants and their products: inflammatory and other signal pathways. *Nutrition and Cancer.*

PINEAPPLE
Amini A, Ehteda A, Masoumi Moghaddam S, Akhter J, Pillai K, Morris DL.(2013) Cytotoxic effects of bromelain in human gastrointestinal carcinoma cell lines (MKN45, KATO-III, HT29-5F12, and HT29-5M21). *Oncology Targets and Therapy*.

Hale LP, Chichlowski M, Trinh CT, Greer PK. (2010) Dietary supplementation with fresh pineapple juice decreases inflammation and colonic neoplasia in IL-10-deficient mice with colitis. *Inflammatory Bowel Disease*.

Romano B, Fasolino I, Pagano E, Capasso R, Pace S, De Rosa G, Milic N, Orlando P, Izzo AA, Borrelli F. (2014) The chemopreventive action of bromelain, from pineapple stem (Ananas comosus L.), on colon carcinogenesis is related to antiproliferative and proapoptotic effects. *Molecular Nutrition & Food Research*.

Sae-Teaw M, Johns J, Johns NP, Subongkot S. (2013) Serum melatonin levels and antioxidant capacities after consumption of pineapple, orange, or banana by healthy male volunteers. *Journal of Pineal Research*.

PLUM
Baliga MS. (2011) Anticancer, chemopreventive and radioprotective potential of black plum (Eugenia jambolana lam.). *Asian Pacific Journal of Cancer Prevention*.

Vizzotto M, Porter W, Byrne D, Cisneros-Zevallos L. (2014) Polyphenols of selected peach and plum genotypes reduce cell viability and inhibit proliferation of breast cancer cells while not affecting normal cells. *Food Chemistry*.

POMEGRANATE
Banerjee N, Kim H, Talcott S, Mertens-Talcott S. (2013) Pomegranate polyphenolics suppressed azoxymethane-induced colorectal aberrant crypt foci and inflammation: possible role of miR-126/VCAM-1 and miR-126/PI3K/AKT/mTOR. *Carcinogenesis*.

Munagala R, Aqil F, Vadhanam MV, Gupta RC. (2013) MicroRNA 'signature' during estrogen-mediated mammary carcinogenesis and its reversal by ellagic acid intervention. *Cancer Letters.*

Nuñez-Sánchez MA, García-Villalba R, Monedero-Saiz T, García-Talavera NV, Gómez-Sánchez MB, Sánchez-Álvarez C, García-Albert AM, Rodríguez-Gil FJ, Ruiz-Marín M, Pastor-Quirante FA, Martínez-Díaz F, Yáñez-Gascón MJ, González-Sarrías A, Tomás-Barberán FA, Espín JC. (2014) Targeted metabolic profiling of pomegranate polyphenols and urolithins in plasma, urine and colon tissues from colorectal cancer patients. *Molecular Nutrition & Food Research.*

Rocha A, Wang L, Penichet M, Martins-Green M. (2012) Pomegranate juice and specific components inhibit cell and molecular processes critical for metastasis of breast cancer. *Breast Cancer Treatment and Research.*

Vicinanza R, Zhang Y, Henning SM, Heber D. (2013) Pomegranate Juice Metabolites, Ellagic Acid and Urolithin A, Synergistically Inhibit Androgen-Independent Prostate Cancer Cell Growth via Distinct Effects on Cell Cycle Control and Apoptosis. *Evidence Based Complementary Alternative Medicine.*

PROTEIN POWDER
de Campos-Ferraz PL, Andrade I, das Neves W, Hangai I, Alves CR, Lancha Jr AH. (2014) An overview of amines as nutritional supplements to counteract cancer cachexia. *Journal of Cachexia, Sarcopenia and Muscle.*

PRUNES
Stacewicz-Sapuntzakis M. (2013) Dried plums and their products: composition and health effects--an updated review. *Critical Reviews of Food Science and Nutrition.*

Yu, MH. (2007) Induction of apoptosis by immature fruits of Prunus salicina Lindl. cv. Soldam in MDA-MB-231 human breast cancer cells. *International Journal of Food Sciences and Nutrition.*

RASPBERRIES
Mallery SR, Tong M, Shumway BS, Curran AE, Larsen PE, Ness GM, Kennedy KS, Blakey GH, Kushner GM, Vickers AM, Han B, Pei P, Stoner GD. (2014) Topical application of a muco-adhesive freeze-dried black raspberry gel induces clinical and histologic regression and reduces loss of heterozygosity events in premalignant oral intraepithelial lesions: results from a multicentered, placebo-controlled clinical trial. *Clinical Cancer Research.*

Munagala R, Aqil F, Vadhanam MV, Gupta RC. (2013) MicroRNA 'signature' during estrogen-mediated mammary carcinogenesis and its reversal by ellagic acid intervention. *Cancer Letters.*

Olsson, ME. (2004). Inhibition of cancer cell proliferation in vitro by fruit and berry extracts and correlations with antioxidant levels. *Journal of Agricultural and Food Chemistry.*

Peiffer DS, Zimmerman NP, Wang LS, Ransom B, Carmella SG, Kuo CT, Siddiqui J, Chen JH, Oshima K, Huang YW, Hecht SS, Stoner GD. (2014) Chemoprevention of esophageal cancer with black raspberries, their component anthocyanins, and a major anthocyanin metabolite, protocatechuic acid. *Cancer Prevention Research (Phila).*

Wang LS, Kuo CT, Stoner K, Yearsley M, Oshima K, Yu J, Huang TH, Rosenberg D, Peiffer D, Stoner G, Huang YW. (2013) Dietary black raspberries modulate DNA methylation in dextran sodium sulfate (DSS)-induced ulcerative colitis. *Carcinogenesis.*

ROSEMARY

Berdowska I, Zieliński B, Fecka I, Kulbacka J, Saczko J, Gamian A. (2013) Cytotoxic impact of phenolics from Lamiaceae species on human breast cancer cells. *Food Chemistry.*

Einbond LS, Wu HA, Kashiwazaki R, He K, Roller M, Su T, Wang X, Goldsberry S. (2012) Carnosic acid inhibits the growth of ER-negative human breast cancer cells and synergizes with curcumin. *Fitoterapia.*

Johnson JJ. (2011) Carnosol: a promising anticancer and anti-inflammatory agent. *Cancer Letters.*

Khuda-Bukhsh AR1, Das S, Saha SK. (2014) Molecular approaches toward targeted cancer prevention with some food plants and their products: inflammatory and other signal pathways. *Nutrition and Cancer.*

Kontogianni VG, Tomic G, Nikolic I, Nerantzaki AA, Sayyad N, Stosic-Grujicic S, Stojanovic I, Gerothanassis IP, Tzakos AG. (2013). Phytochemical profile of Rosmarinus officinalis and Salvia officinalis extracts and correlation to their antioxidant and antiproliferative activity. *Food Chemistry.*

Ngo SN, Williams DB, Head RJ. (2011) Rosemary and cancer prevention: preclinical perspectives. *Critical Reviews in Food Science and Nutrition.*

Park KW, Kundu J, Chae IG, Kim DH, Yu MH, Kundu JK, Chun KS. (2014) Carnosol induces apoptosis through generation of ROS and inactivation of STAT3 signaling in human colon cancer HCT116 cells. *International Journal of Oncology.*

Yesil-Celiktas O, Sevimli C, Bedir E, Vardar-Sukan F. (2010) Inhibitory effects of rosemary extracts, carnosic acid and rosmarinic acid on the growth of various human cancer cell lines. *Plant Foods and Human Nutrition.*

SPEARMINT
Yu TW, Xu M, Dashwood RH. (2004) Antimutagenic activity of spearmint. *Environmental and Molecular Mutagenesis.*

SPINACH
Khuda-Bukhsh AR, Das S, Saha SK. (2014) Molecular approaches toward targeted cancer prevention with some food plants and their products: inflammatory and other signal pathways. *Nutrition and Cancer.*

Mizushina Y, Hada T, Yoshida H. (2012) In vivo antitumor effect of liposomes with sialyl Lewis X including monogalactosyl diacylglycerol, a replicative DNA polymerase inhibitor, from spinach. *Oncology Reports.*

STRAWBERRIES
Giampieri F, Alvarez-Suarez JM, Battino M. (2014) Strawberry and Human Health: Effects beyond Antioxidant Activity. *Journal of Agricultural and Food Chemistry.*

Munagala R, Aqil F, Vadhanam MV, Gupta RC. (2013) MicroRNA 'signature' during estrogen-mediated mammary carcinogenesis and its reversal by ellagic acid intervention. *Cancer Letters.*

Seeram, NP. (2006) Blackberry, black raspberry, blueberry, cranberry, red raspberry, and strawberry extracts inhibit growth and stimulate apoptosis of human cancer cells in vitro. *Journal of Agricultural and Food Chemistry.*

Somasagara RR, Hegde M, Chiruvella KK, Musini A, Choudhary B, Raghavan SC. (2012) Extracts of strawberry fruits induce intrinsic pathway of apoptosis in breast cancer cells and inhibit tumor progression in mice. *PLoS One*.

Syed DN, Adhami VM, Khan MI, Mukhtar H. (2013) Inhibition of Akt/mTOR signaling by the dietary flavonoid fisetin. *Anticancer Agents Medicinal Chemistry*.

TANGERINES
Baek SH, Kim SM, Nam D, Lee JH, Ahn KS, Choi SH, Kim SH, Shim BS, Chang IM, Ahn KS. (2012) Antimetastatic effect of nobiletin through the down-regulation of CXC chemokine receptor type 4 and matrix metallopeptidase-9. *Pharmaceutical Biology*.

Dong Y, Cao A, Shi J, Yin P, Wang L, Ji G, Xie J, Wu D. (2014) Tangeretin, a citrus polymethoxyflavonoid, induces apoptosis of human gastric cancer AGS cells through extrinsic and intrinsic signaling pathways. *Oncology Reports*.

Lakshmi A, Subramanian S. (2014) Chemotherapeutic effect of tangeretin, a polymethoxylated flavone studied in 7, 12-dimethylbenz(a)anthracene induced mammary carcinoma in experimental rats. *Biochimie*.

Lee, CJ. (2009) Hesperidin suppressed proliferations of both human breast cancer and androgen-dependent prostate cancer cells. *Phytotherapy Research*.

TART CHERRIES
Kang SY, Seeram NP, Nair MG, Bourquin LD. (2003) Tart cherry anthocyanins inhibit tumor development in Apc(Min) mice and reduce proliferation of human colon cancer cells. *Cancer Letters*.

Martin KR, Wooden A. (2012) Tart Cherry Juice Induces Differential Dose-Dependent Effects on Apoptosis, But Not Cellular Proliferation, in MCF-7 Human Breast Cancer Cells. *Journal of Medicinal Food.*

Traustadóttir T, Davies SS, Stock AA, Su Y, Heward CB, Roberts LJ 2nd, Harman SM. (2009) Tart cherry juice decreases oxidative stress in healthy older men and women. *Journal of Nutrition.*

TOMATO
Bhuvaneswari V, & Nagini S. (2005) Lycopene: a review of its potential as an anticancer agent. *Current Medicinal Therapy Anticancer Agents.*

Khuda-Bukhsh AR, Das S, Saha SK. (2014) Molecular approaches toward targeted cancer prevention with some food plants and their products: inflammatory and other signal pathways. *Nutrition and Cancer.*

Mignone, LI. (2009) Dietary carotenoids and the risk of invasive breast cancer. *International Journal of Cancer.*

Thomson, CA. (2007) Plasma and dietary carotenoids are associated with reduced oxidative stress in women previously treated for breast cancer. *Cancer Epidemiology, Biomarkers and Prevention.*

TURMERIC
Alfano CM, Imayama I, Neuhouser ML, Kiecolt-Glaser JK, Smith AW, Meeske K, McTiernan A, Bernstein L, Baumgartner KB, Ulrich CM, Ballard-Barbash R. (2012) Fatigue, inflammation, and ω-3 and ω-6 fatty acid intake among breast cancer survivors. *Journal of Clinical Oncology.*

Chen J, Wang FL, Chen WD. (2014) Modulation of apoptosis-related cell signaling pathways by curcumin as a strategy to inhibit tumor progression. *Molecular Biology Reports*.

Liu H, Liu YZ, Zhang F, Wang HS, Zhang G, Zhou BH, Zuo YL, Cai SH, Bu XZ, Du J. (2014) Identification of potential pathways involved in the induction of cell cycle arrest and apoptosis by a new 4-arylidene curcumin analogue T63 in lung cancer cells: a comparative proteomic analysis. *Molecular Biosystems*.

Lv J, Shao Q, Wang H, Shi H, Wang T, Gao W, Song B, Zheng G, Kong B, Qu X. (2013) Effects and mechanisms of curcumin and basil polysaccharide on the invasion of SKOV3 cells and dendritic cells. *Molecular Medicine Reports*.

Xia, Y. (2007) The potentiation of curcumin on insulin-like growth factor-1 action in MCF-7 human breast carcinoma cells. *Life Sciences*.

VANILLA
Khuda-Bukhsh AR, Das S, Saha SK. (2014) Molecular approaches toward targeted cancer prevention with some food plants and their products: inflammatory and other signal pathways. *Nutrition and Cancer*.

Lirdprapamongkol K, Sakurai H, Kawasaki N, Choo MK, Saitoh Y, Aozuka Y, Singhirunnusorn P, Ruchirawat S, Svasti J, Saiki I. (2005) Vanillin suppresses in vitro invasion and in vivo metastasis of mouse breast cancer cells. *European Journal of Pharmaceutical Sciences*.

Lirdprapamongkol K, Sakurai H, Suzuki S, Koizumi K, Prangsaengtong O, Viriyaroj A, Ruchirawat S, Svasti J, Saiki I. (2010) Vanillin enhances TRAIL-induced apoptosis in cancer cells through inhibition of NF-kappaB activation. *In Vivo*.

Shi ZY, Li YQ, Kang YH, Hu GQ, Huang-fu CS, Deng JB, Liu B. (2012) Piperonal ciprofloxacin hydrazone induces growth arrest and apoptosis of human hepatocarcinoma SMMC-7721 cells. *Journal of the Chinese Pharmacological Society.*

WATERMELON
Agca CA, Tuzcu M, Gencoglu H, Akdemir F, Ali S, Sahin K, Kucuk O. (2012) Lycopene counteracts the hepatic response to 7,12-dimethylbenz[a]anthracene by altering the expression of Bax, Bcl-2, caspases, and oxidative stress biomarkers. *Pharmaceutical Biology.*

Bhuvaneswari V, & Nagini S. (2005) Lycopene: a review of its potential as an anticancer agent. *Current Medicinal Chemistry Anticancer Agents.*

Li-Xinli, Xu-Jiuhong. (2014) Meta-analysis of the association between dietary lycopene intake and ovarian cancer risk in postmenopausal women. *Scientific Reports.*

Mignone L I. (2009) Dietary carotenoids and the risk of invasive breast cancer. *International Journal of Cancer.*

Takata Y, Xiang YB, Yang G, Li H, Gao J, Cai H, Gao YT, Zheng W, Shu XO. (2013) Intakes of fruits, vegetables, and related vitamins and lung cancer risk: results from the Shanghai Men's Health Study (2002-2009). *Nutrition and Cancer.*

WHITE TEA
Bhardwaj J, Chaudhary N, Seo HJ, Kim MY, Shin TS, Kim JD. (2014) Immunomodulatory effect of tea saponin in immune T-cells and T-lymphoma cells via regulation of Th1, Th2 immune response and MAPK/ERK2 signaling pathway. *Immunopharmacology and Immunotoxicology.*

Gardener H, Rundek T, Wright CB, Elkind MS, Sacco RL. (2013) Coffee and tea consumption are inversely associated with mortality in a multiethnic urban population. *Journal of Nutrition.*

WILD BLUEBERRIES
Dinstel RR, Cascio J, Koukel S. (2013) The antioxidant level of Alaska's wild berries: high, higher and highest. *International Journal of Circumpolar Health.*

Wilms LC, Boots AW, de Boer VC, Maas LM, Pachen DM, Gottschalk RW, Ketelslegers HB, Godschalk RW, Haenen GR, van Schooten FJ, Kleinjans JC. (2007) Impact of multiple genetic polymorphisms on effects of a 4-week blueberry juice intervention on ex vivo induced lymphocytic DNA damage in human volunteers. *Carcinogenesis.*

Acknowledgments

The author also wishes to acknowledge the following supporters:

Linda Landkammer, who has read and edited every single word in each of my manuscripts providing practical ideas and gentle critiques that improve the usability of my books.

Matias Booth, my culinary consultant, who applied his innate ability to combine intense flavors in winning combinations to many of these recipes.

Abigail Gehring, my new editor at Skyhorse Publishing, for her vision and appreciation of the value of whole foods nutrition.

Tony Lyons at Skyhorse Publishing, a special thank you to you for making this book happen.

Anne Rierson at Frontier Co-op, thank you for supplying my recipe development team with our favorite Frontier artisan quality herbs, spices, and teas.

Tami Elwin at Zico, thank you for the delicious coconut water that has gone into thousands of medicinal smoothies in my test kitchen.

Cassidy Stockton at Bob's Red Mill, thank you for supplying the product that has supported the development of healing recipes in dozens of my books.

Nancy England of the Wild Blueberry Association of North America and Wyman's of Maine, thank you for the luscious wild blueberries.

Michael Wray at Mariner for the MacGourmet Nutrition Analysis Software.

Karie Duff at Epicurean, thank you for the innovative kitchen tools—silicone spatulas and pressed paper cutting boards.

Also a big thank you to the following companies for providing product support: Tribest, VitaMix, Ninja Blender, Blendtec, Omega, OXO, Fronteir, Cuisinart, Epicurean, Northwest Wild Foods, Bormioli Rocco, and So Delicious.

About the Author

Daniella Chace, MSc, CN, is a clinical nutritionist and educator. She is an expert in personalized medical nutrition therapy, with an emphasis in toxicology, epigenetics, human microbial ecology, and orthomolecular applications in disease management.

She is the author of over twenty nutrition books and the host of NPR's *Nutrition Matters*. She lives in Port Townsend, Washington, where she sees clients in her private practice and develops recipes that support healing.

Learn more at daniellachace.com.

Index